The Accidental Diet

From *Fugly* to *fox*

By:

Alicia Hunter

Edited by:

Amy Hunter-Dutta

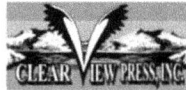

ClearView Press Inc.

Palm Coast FL

The Accidental Diet   *From Fugly to Fox*

By Alicia Hunter

Copyright © 2011 by ClearView Press Inc.

ISBN 978-1-935795-88-9

LCCN 2011940497

Content Editor: Amy Hunter-Dutta

Cover Design by: Stefon Miller

ClearView Press Inc.

PO Box 353431

Palm Coast FL 32135-3431

www.clearviewpressinc.com

Printed in the United States of America

DEDICATION

To my beautiful, undyingly influential son, Hunter. Some people live an entire life and seem to barely touch many beyond their immediate realm. Others are here on earth so briefly, yet their flame burns on and on…

I have two distinct lives: one before I met Hunter, one after. The one before was filled with a lot of happy times, but a ton of angst, questioning of self-worth, pettiness, and sadness. Little did I know what pain truly was, until Hunter was here, then inexplicably taken.

Fortunately for me, my "after" life has overflowed with amazing, incredible people and the opportunities they have brought to me. Many I feel have been sent to me personally by my Angel, to guide me and assist me, with nothing asked in return. My hope for the readers of this book is that they find, like I did, that life is truly beautiful – meant to be lived to its fullest and surrounded by positive people. If there are things you are not satisfied with about your own life, remember that *you* have the power to change anything – to turn negatives into positives. Whatever your lot in life, build something on it. Squeeze every ounce of life out of each day, remember how lucky you are to be here, and always pay it forward, and you, too, will be richly blessed.

Thank you Hunter, for teaching mommy what was missing from her life. My baby butterfly – thanks for teaching me how to spread my own wings and fly ☺

SHOUT-OUTS

Wow. So many fabulous peeps to thank, I'm not sure where to begin…so – in order of appearance, here is the cast of characters in my life that made this book possible:

Dad & Mom –

For their undying support – these are the type of parents that if I or any of my siblings wanted to do anything in life, be anything – the sky was the limit. I am sure that if I'd said I wanted to grow up and be a serial killer, they'd have said, "Yay, you! Just go out there, then, and be the best darn serial killer that you can be!" So, yeah – my heroes – THANKS you two! Without you, I wouldn't be here. Or anywhere, quite frankly.

Amy –

Thank YOU for bothering to get a Masters in English! Thanks for being a perpetually amazing scholar, so I could just cozy up with a gallon of chocolate chip mint and practically not finish high school…hey, also, if this book does well, I can finally settle up with you on the hundreds of dollars I must owe you (one quarter at a time) for fetching MY lazy ass glass upon glass of ice water when we were kids. What a slothy brat I was! Sorry about that. I owe you! Thanks for being my late-night buddy, watching 1980's SNL episodes….remember- we Aren't Really Sistahs, but we Are Really Ugly…thanks for, in fact, possessing an inner monologue…☺ Thanks also for your amazing muffin recipe additions!

Ah, Rebekah. Rebekah, Rebekah, Rebekah…the inspiration for thinking I, too, could ask Mike King and ClearView Press to even look at my book. I know the only reason they did is because Motherhood Is Easy ROCKED! Thanks for fluffing up your coattails and allowing me to go for a tiny ride…and thanks also for allowing me to continuously rattle on like only I can do, while I can hear you officially "powering down" over the phone. "I hope I haven't bored you… Ka-POW!!!" Think of me whenever the schnecken beckons…

Carrie –
Thanks for allowing me to shower you with my Idea Files.

Mattster & Evan -
Matt, thanks for NOTHING. Tee hee – no, really - thanks in advance for reading this book…if even just this page so you can see your name in print..;) Evan – thanks for being a perpetual inspiration by just being you, and for making me laugh with your YouTube finds…honey badger don't care….:)

Andre, Derek, Annabel, Rollie, Elsa, Finley – thanks for letting me borrow your mommies!
Trevor & Dog – you also!
Sabrin, Jeff, Morris & Jenny – thanks for being awesome better halves to my sibs ☺

Hunter –

My inspiration – the little-big dude who, through your short time in my arms, taught me how to LIVE. My prayer is that since I couldn't keep you here, I roll out a legacy in your honor of guiding many to see what really matters in this world. 11-11.

Ashley & Hazy –

Thanks for loving Sponge Bob, Power Rangers and I-Carly enough so that mommy could spend hours on this book instead of playing with you! I will make it up to you very soon at The Magic Kingdom, where we will spend hours winding our way through sweaty, fanny-pack-wearing tourists, slurp overpriced yet delicious mickey-pops, and watch an embarrassing amount of fireworks…I Love You More.

James – hon, what can I say – without your help (and especially your affinity for cooking!), this book would not have been possible, because without you, we wouldn't have had Hunter, and therefore the inspiration for all things amazing that we have to be thankful for. Thanks for pulling double-duty on the parenting front – forever grateful.

Debbie L!

Honey! I can't LIVE without you! Your never-ending help, shoulder to vent on, cry on, laugh on – Lucy & Ethel got Nothin' on us! Just wait – Richard Widmark's grapefruit tree? Chocolate conveyor belt? Child's play!! Thanks for all your help with m'kiddos, so they didn't have to be completely raised by wolves…D-Lo – the incredible shrinking man without even running over a gypsy (allegedly ☺) – thanks for lending me so much time with your wife; when you weren't using her, I was ☺

Alexandra, Shane & Madison L –
A trio of fabulous kiddos! Thanks for being big brothers and sisters to Ash & Hazy! Alex – you in fact inspired me to get busy reaching out to young ladies to encourage kindness! Thanks for providing me with insight I would not have otherwise had…Love you guys! I hope my kidlets grow up to be as wonderful as you! ☺

VIVIAN G –
What can I say, my sister-from-another-mister? I treasure you and your endless energy and dedication !!! THANK YOU for so many things, too many to list! I can't wait until you teach me how to properly Lombada, or whatever that dance is called….:) and then we shall go out for pancakes and Veuve!!

Matthew B –
(that fortuitous cab ride from The Hotel Belmont – who knew we'd have more fun Leaving the Superbowl than actually attending it!) – and we've only just begun…I look forward to many rolls, rolls, rolls in ze hayyy with YOU!

Jackie S –

Babe! How cool are you?? More gorgeous on the inside than out, as if that's even possible – but it is! Rock on with your brilliant, foxy, kind self. ☺

Xenia S-

Honey – keep walking into things so I can lash you always! Thanks for making me laugh and being such a rockin' girlfriend! ☺
Vincenza!!
Oh, no she di-int! Oh YES SHE DIT!!!
Girrrllll – where WOULD I be without you and your magical smokey eye?? Hideous, for one thing. I look forward to many many MANY Green Room Fox & Green Room "L" sessions with you and da gang!

Sindy with an "S" –
You ROCKED my hair for the book photos! And you just ROCK in general! Thanks babe!

Ashleigh B –
!!!! Thank YOU for being my sounding board, for believing I could do this book, and for all the other ways you are a true girlfriend! I look forward to many future chin-wags and lots and lots of LAUGHS! You are a true superwoman and an inspiration that we can, in fact, do it All! And always remember – if you flush a goldfish and no one's there to see it, did it really happen?

Don S –

What can I say? Without your encouragement and support, this book wouldn't have been anything more than a Word Doc sitting in a laptop file…THANK YOU thank you thank you thank you infinity!

To Mike King, Bobbie, Cindy, CVP – thanks a million for believing in me! Let's rock this book!

Shout-outs to:

Dr. Susie P. – first, for literally saving my life and Hunter's life, and for encouraging me to give Ashley hers…for inspiring me as the fabulous mother / physician that you are, and for giving me that extra time that I know you can never give, but always do. Thanks from the bottom of my heart. I have the family I have because of you and your hopeful attitude and direction…grateful to you always.

Beth V – ah, Beth…my long-time supporter, laugh-buddy, and fellow-lover of all things Irreverent…Too many things to thank you for…you know what they are, anyway…so THANKS & love ya! Now, if I can only get you to change your voter registration back…ha!

Marc & Elena Finer, for always believing in me, especially when it was bleak! Two special people ☺

Uncle Ted & Aunt Mary & Erika – for being so fun to be around, and your inspiration through example ☺

Aunt Patti, Uncle CJ, Kimmie & Brandi – for being such amazing people, for the terrific memories, and Aunt Patti – for inspiring me to channel my inner go-go dancer when required! ☺

Didi & Mimi – I cannot imagine how ragged my grammar would be without Arb-Dib! And how much faster those Scrabble games could've gone…☺

Aunt Joanie & Uncle Vinnie, Steve, Kenny & Deb- for all those ice cream cones, introducing me to lunch meat, Foreigner, flashlight tag & bats! Xxoo you guys!

Dr. Jill W – THANKS FRIEND for believing in me and making me think this not only could, but Should happen! Love you always!! And thanks of course for my face-full of Vitamin "B" and all things hyaluronic! Tee hee…

Betty N – for your enduring friendship and soulful advice – and the HAIR!!! I'd be lost without you for all the ways in which you've enriched my life.☺

Andrea M – thank you for always being there as a friend – and, of course, the perfect tan!

Jennifer K – thanks for saying "oh! You have a book??" ☺

Kerri W – for giving me great opportunities, many of which led to the fire in my belly to get this party started! Little P is a lucky dude ☺ you & TJ enjoy every second! I know you will…

Tobin S – for lending me a tiny part of your brilliant brain. Don't worry, I left you some!

Mike B – for watching this all unfold, and for your biz intellect. THANKS!

Pachi L – for being such a beautiful, teaching soul. Love you more! BESITOS

Richie R – for keeping my brain sharp and therefore somewhat witty ☺

Marsia T – for being YOU! Remember – NEVER open your own door or your own wallet! Rock it South Philly-Style!

Lauren T – for being your amazing, foxy self…and for voting the right way!

Emily G – for your insight and surprisingly irreverent spirit – I guess that's what happens when you're married to a Kennedy…

Lisa B – thanks for showing me how to drop it like it's hot, and for just being "what IS she?" haaaaa

David C – for renewing my faith in friendships old and new, and for being as hopeful as I try to be! Oh, and thanks also for the illustrious tour of Claire's wine cellar/gym…

Claire DK – girlfriend! Adore you then, now, and in the future! We've got lots to do…

Rob F – thanks for being my dance partner at U2 – we rocked the house, huh?

Carla – for your undying friendship and faith in the both of us!

Kimmie GM – love you, lady! We WILL Shoot!

Sue HA – again, friend old & new – truly in my irreverent thoughts…

DISCLAIMER

I am not a doctor, nor have I ever played one on TV. But I did consult a registered dietician when forming the menu plans in this book.

The author (that's me) and the publisher specifically disclaim any and all liability arising directly or indirectly from the use or application of any information contained in this book. And as always, before you start any new eating program, you should consult a health care professional.

TABLE OF CONTENTS

PROLOGUE

This book isn't for everyone. For example, it's not for people who feel like they have no need for encouragement, or for those who've felt like hot stuff from the ages of 9-15, or who have always felt like Prom Queen, or who can open an invitation to any event at any given time and go "Hell, yeah! I can't *wait* to attend that class reunion / family function / party! It's next week, but I look exactly like I want to look *today,* and in fact, if the event *were* today, I have no problem walking out the door right *now* because there's nothing I'd want to improve upon in the looks department! I look darn good in everything hanging in my closet – so good, in fact, that it's going to be impossible to find what looks the best on me! Woooo Hoooo!"

This book is for anyone who's ever felt like they were a Fugly – slang for Fat Ugly. Hence the subtitle…

Or combinations thereof. Frettys or Thuglys are welcome to read on, also.

When I was recently in Victoria's Secret (yeah, her secret is that her fragrances smell like Early American Strip-Joint and her corsets would make Scarlett O'Hara beg for mercy)…

Ah, I digress. Get used to it, if you plan to continue reading. It's my writing style. But I do have something to say, so if you can switch gears fairly easily, then I'm for you…

Any-who, when I was recently in Vicky's Secret, I was measured by a "brassiere specialist" who clocked me at a 32-C. You talkin' to me? I instinctively turned around and bumped into a sluttilydressed mannequin with such force that her right arm twisted behind her and fell off, because I was trying to see just who the hell the "BS" could possibly have been talking to.

Shockingly, it was me. Me?! I still have difficulty registering my much smaller size, having spent 30 years at least 30 pounds overweight, and only the past 6 years in this new bod. Reconciling an enviable dress-size with a formerly-chubby soul is tricky business. I'm still figuring that part out. But I can assure you, it's well worth the confusion.

I am the girl who used to stand on my bathroom scale, positioned close enough to the bathroom counter that I could rest one arm on it and put part of my weight on that arm, just to see what a number much lower might actually look like...

I am the mommy who, when my kids openly and giddily hopped up onto the grocery store scale upon exiting with a cartful, scowled and sharply yelled, "Come ON, we need to GET GOING!" just so they wouldn't be able to force me onto the scale, thinking it was all in good fun...

I am the woman who used to check out other women, not to see about their style or covet their shoes, but to look longingly at their toned bodies, slender arms, great posture – and ask myself "how does she do it? How does she look like that? What's her secret to looking like she's got it going on? She probably lives on a treadmill and eats kale all day long! Because that "look" must be impossible to achieve!"

I am the friend who always rocked the great personality. Because I couldn't rock a bikini.

One day, I received an attitude adjustment and dropped the common albatross, and it was too easy and too impactful not to share how. If you're ready to do the same, then read on, friend.

You probably bought this book because there is something about yourself that you don't like. Maybe you feel like I did…a Fugly Duck, the swan inside of you just waiting to get out. This is either for aesthetic reasons, health reasons – or most likely both.

This isn't the first weight-loss book you've bought, borrowed or maybe even stolen. Geez, I wish I had a dollar for every copy of *Atkins New Diet Revolution* I angrily threw into the garbage can and buried under a doughnut wrapper.

Here are some questions you may want to ask yourself before reading this book:

1. Have you tried other diets and failed?
2. Do you avoid exercise?
3. Do you think you're a different person on the inside than the body you wear on the outside?
4. Do you feel like you don't want to meet people because this isn't how you really look?
5. Do you think about your weight constantly?
6. Have you received a poor medical report or has your doctor cautioned you of health risks associated with being overweight?
7. Do you go to bed every night trying to land on which diet you're going to try next, and do you wake up each morning with renewed hope, only to go off the diet within days of starting it?

8. Once you "fall off your diet", do you eat whatever you want for the rest of that day / week until the following Monday so you can "start over" then?

9. Do you closely associate your happiness with being slimmer and self-loathing with being heavy?

10. Do you have people in your past that you don't want to run into while you're at your present weight because you don't want them to see you now?

11. Do you avoid activities because you don't have proper clothes for them?

12. Do you avoid activities/invitations because you are unhappy with your appearance?

13. Do you wish there was a magic pill that could make you lose weight?

14. Do you feel like you'd do anything to lose weight?

15. Do you think you're in a relationship (or previous relationships) where you're putting up with someone you wouldn't have to if you had the body you wanted?

16. Are you concerned with how your self-disappointment affects your children?

17. Do you hope your own children won't have to worry about their weight later in life?

18. Are you inactive and therefore don't participate with your children due to your weight?

19. Have you been overlooked for a job or a promotion due to your looks?

20. Are you unhappy with the way you are aging?

21. Have you seen a friend who looks spectacular and now you feel inadequate and want to make a change in yourself?

22. Do you avoid wearing shorts / short sleeves / bathing suits in warm weather and this draws attention from others and makes you uncomfortable?

23. Do you have several different sizes of clothes in your house?

24. Do you avoid cameras?

25. If someone takes out their camera in your vicinity, do you immediately reach for the nearest pillow, small dog or newborn baby to hold in front of you, thereby blocking the camera's view?

26. If you can't avoid the camera, are you miffed at the photographer?

27. Do you break into relatives'/friends' homes at night to steal back fat pictures of yourself?

28. If you received an invitation to a reunion or similar event today in the mail, would you immediately panic about your weight?

29. Do you eat for reasons other than hunger?

30. Are you sincerely ready to break this cycle of eating because you aren't the weight you want to be?

If you answered yes to any or all of these…take heart, my child, you've come to the right place. Let me show you how I lost 55 pounds and kept it off, without dieting, without deprivation. If only I had known this was so easy, I would've lived a much happier life and avoided decades of self-disgust because of my weight.

I hope that you found this read to be not only entertaining, but useful! If you've never met me, you cannot know just how sincerely this has been written. I truly never imagined in my wildest dreams that I would weigh as an adult what I weighed in fifth grade, after having gained and lost hundreds of pounds over 30 years! If you think feeling great in your own skin is life-changing – guess what? You're 100000% right. You couldn't be right-er.

I promise you that if I could incorporate the "nickel and dime" changes detailed in this book, and literally transport myself from an insecure, exercise-hating, ice-cream-sucking weakling into a strong, healthy woman, not afraid to step on a public, grocery store scale – then there is noooo reason you can't, too.

And don't wait til Monday. That's ridiculous and you know it. You're not on death row, so stop eating like an inmate having their final meal on any or every given Sunday, pretending that you're going to "start your diet tomorrow." I started mid-day on a Wednesday in August 2006, and you cannot imagine the light bulb that went off after the first week – heyyyyy, this isn't rocket science. It's not tricky, or expensive. It's combining all the sensible, small changes that add up to consistent, permanent weight loss. That's it. No mystery. Just common sense, people! You owe it to yourself to have the existence that's rightfully yours for the taking.

Start today. Your life is waiting.

CHAPTER ONE

My Story: The Good, the Bad & the Fugly

Together, let's take a light-hearted journey through the Valley of the Diets. Together, let's see how much money and time we've wasted, to remind ourselves that we're not doing that again.....Come on, it'll be fun! I'll start, beginning chronologically with when I myself did them, and why:

The Dawn of Chub

1977 – Age 10. This is when I first realized I was, um, pasty and also chunkier than my peers. Sigh. Upon asking my mom if I was fat and being told that I was not fat but that I could try some mascara (???), I decided to try snacking on dog biscuits between meals rather than on actual food. These were portable and fit nicely inside my winter coat. I also took to eating shredded tissues which I kept in with the Milk Bones, kind of an early spin on trail mix. What it lacked in flavor it conquered in texture. While I don't condone this type of behavior, it's mostly because I'm uncertain of the caloric content more so than that I'm keeping you from a quite filling snack (which it definitely is). After all, aren't you counting on me to keep your calories in check? Just doing my job.

I recall now that when I read books, I would zero in on the parts that detailed food. Much like skipping through the dialogue to get to the action when watching porn, I would seek out, read and re-read descriptions of meals or mere mention of the word "snack." Nancy

1

Drew and Ned having sandwiches – ooh! Dinah the Cook making tea and cookies for Nan and Bert Bobbsey - ahhhh. I remember one particular ghost story that I read not for the fear factor but because of the description at one point of a character going into the kitchen and slathering butter on a crust of bread….I think the kid was poor, and the author was stressing "crust" to denote having the shittiest part of the bread, but since I like things crunchy, I remember just being, well, turned on by this passage. See, I even remember it now.

This year also heralded Charlie's Angels to my wide eyes. Now, that's what girls are supposed to look like!!! Sexy, long-haired, skinny and tan. I desperately begged for a dime whenever we went to Woolworth's so I could invest in Angel trading cards. But who was I kidding, I wanted the gum - in all its powdery cardboard glory - in my mouth, just as much as I wanted the cards. And I pored over each Angel card, never using my stickers, saving them for Some Day.

The neighborhood girls stopped playing Barbies that summer and instead played Charlie's Angels. I quietly awaited my role assignment. With my new Dorothy Hamill wedge 'do, I knew I'd have to be Sabrina – retrospectively, how I would've gladly accepted that role were I not told "Alicia. You Will Be Bosley."

It was also during this summer that we took our annual family vacation to Kentucky, to my dad's hometown. I had gotten a blue t-shirt with the infamous Farrah Fawcett Majors red bathing suit poster ironed-on to it, and I wasn't often seen without it. My dad took me to the Dollar General one day, to buy jeans and probably some potted meat. A lady of about 117 stopped my dad and exclaimed full-drawl,

"Wayyall, Wayyyyne! Howww R Yew!!!??? And Who is This Youung Maayannn with you???"

My dad stammered, "This is Lisha, my eldest daughter." I don't know if any words were spoken after that; I assume they were, but my ears filled up from the inside with invisible cotton and I'm sure I blacked out. It's possible I slammed into a pyramid display of pecan logs and plastic pinwheels, but I'm not certain. Funny what we remember.

Bummer Camp

1978- Ah, summer camp. To this day, I don't understand the attraction, nor will I ever, ever send my kids away to one. Unless they happen to be really, really great looking and slender when they are between the ages of 9 and 13, I would rather cover them with honey and tie them to ant hills – it would be less painful.

It wasn't that it was summer camp, or that it was Bible camp. It had nothing at all to do with camp, but rather, I was just too unappealing-looking to be in attendance. Not that the other girls were beauty queens, but to me they were. I would just sit on my wooden bunk, staring at them as they flipped their long straight hair, with their tiny gym shorts loosely fitting around their legs and size Small camp tee. I remember checking out my own legs, and discovering that if I were doing anything but standing still, my thighs did weird things. When I sat, they were marshmallowy trunks that melded together into one seamless slab of milkiness. When I walked, my thighs would move kind of on their own, gelatin-like, or at least it seemed that way

3

to me. For a time, I tried to walk without bending my knees at all, so as to create less fluctuation in their movement, but I suppose I looked kind of Frankenstein-ish, because I remember drawing more than a few stares, and some counselors asked me if I had hurt myself on the Slip n' Slide. So I meekly started walking regular again, dismayed that my attempt to stabilize my gluts had instead drawn more attention. Sigh.

If the camp outfits weren't bad enough, there was the pool. Yes, a community pool. A public pool. The kind of pool that inevitably has cheerful signs that say, "Shower Before Entering" and, "Welcome To Our Ool. Notice There's No "P" In "Pool"....Let's Keep It That Way!" The other kids would sometimes not even wear a shirt over their bathing suit! Me, I would layer. And usually went in the pool that way, painfully aware that I was spilling over and out of my suit no matter what size we bought. Just as sausage casing cannot contain the filling if there are openings in the casing, you can't get arms and legs into a bathing suit *without* openings. So you see my dilemma…if only I could've gotten my dimply hands on a wetsuit.

I assume some fellow campers thought I was a leper, an actual Old Testament throw-back. Especially since it *was* Bible camp, we were all acutely aware that this shit can happen, even sometimes to people we know.

Then there was the Fun Activity of doing Jazzercise routines for Show Day. Our group's was to Michael Jackson's *PYT*. I remember being grateful that at least my calves were covered ankle to knee in leg warmer, and I mused how my entire body would look if I pulled the leg

4

warmer all the way up to my leotard crotch. I did try this in the privacy of my own room, but decided against its off-label use.

My diet during this dreamy summer consisted of the following: strictly junk food. I would not eat anything that constituted "real food," like fruits, vegetables, meat or chicken. Instead, I opted only to consume foods that came in a wrapper, which were easily obtained from the camp commissary, for a price. My thought was that since food-food, like you'd eat on a plate, looked bigger, it must make me fatter than smaller, individually-wrapped food. Some days, I would use my entire daily punch-card by late afternoon and then would be ravenous until the next morning, having exhausted my candy bar and potato chip high. Had I known what they were, I would've gladly traded sexual favors for additional snacks, without shame.

The Need For Speed

1979- Age 12. Ah, what a magical age…not really. If you happen to be an awkward, overweight and acutely self-conscious girl, it's actually a rather shitty age.

Enter TV, Well, the *TV Guide* to be exact. I would read it cover-to-cover. I recall being angry when they redid the pages and the shades of gray in the little channel-ID boxes was different. I'm attracted to familiarity, I suppose. In the middle of the *TV Guide*, next to the ballsy dare that you Draw Tippy and mail it in to see if you could be accepted to a Prestigious Art Institute, there was an ad for Diet Pills. *Diet Pills?* Pray tell??? You could eat something that made you skinny??? I couldn't get to a stamp and an envelope fast enough. That

Sunday in church, I volunteered to help clean up after communion for two reasons: one, so I could gobble down the leftover white bread cubes and grape juice that represented the body and blood of Christ, not to be closer to the Lord, but because I was starving; and two, so I could take petty cash from the refreshments jar in the rectory kitchen for my budding drug habit. That night, I taped $15.00 cash to a recipe card with my return address plastered across it. I then met the mailman day after day for about three weeks, knowing that I would need to intercept the box lest any nosy busy-body grownups try to hone in on my skinny plans because they wanted me to stay grotesque.

I never had a Christmas before or since that I anticipated as much as opening that box. Out spilled a white jar that contained capsules that looked like they contained teeny gumballs, and were called some long word that started with A. One can only assume now that they were straight-up amphetamines of unknown origin. I marvel at all the stop-gap measures that are in play these days to prevent prepubescents from ordering speed through the mail. Ah, the 1970's.

I ingested a pill a day for about a month, since that's all I had. I don't remember how they made me feel or whether they made me eat less, more, or if I lost any weight. All I know is after a month, I was still chubby and pale and still enjoyed nothing more than holing up in the family room on a perfectly gorgeous day to watch back-to-back Brady Bunch episodes while feasting on white bread rolled into little balls that I made myself.

The Hundred and Two Pounder

1980- Age 13. This was the year that held promise. Some ladies at my mom's church were all noticing at once that they needed to lose weight, so they started a kind of diet cult. Mom told me they decided to eschew bread in favor of using iceberg lettuce leaves. They began rolling pretty much everything they ate in a lettuce leaf. I'd watch when she had friends over - meat loaf slices, tuna, whatever. They'd be in a little row, smoothing down their leaves while humming along to a Peter, Paul & Mary 8-track, tamping down the filling, and then carefully rolling up the leaf and sealing it with a dollop of mayo. I do not know for a fact but I can now speculate that what the anti-bread cult didn't realize is that this idea was most likely dreamed up by a huge pot-smoker, maybe even as a cruel joke. I would never tell them that. Me? I did try the non-bread thing for a little while, but I don't think it made much difference. Ya can't stick lettuce in a toaster.

This was also the year that my worst fear came true: my private realization of my heft became public. Apparently, school administrators are masochists, as are their Satanic minions, the school nurses. I picture them getting together over cauldrons of steaming humanity, pitching ideas around of how best to humiliate the most vulnerable among us – teenagers. One way they achieved this was by weighing us all in a room together at the start of the school year. My last name was mid-alphabet, so I got to hear everyone's weight before leaving the room to wait out in the hall for the rest of the class. Hey,

7

that's cool – only classmates with last names ending in H through Z would know my shame….no biggie.

"Andy Downs…… 84"

"David Comstock….. 86"

"Julie Dillerd…….72"

"Elizabeth Gunther…..69"

"Alicia Hunter…..102"

Billy Strawderman caught my eye as I shuffled out of the room, painfully aware of the number difference between everyone and me, even the boys. "Hey, Hundred-And-Two Pounder!!!" he yelled to me. No one else said anything. I cannot blame Billy, because he was bestowed with such material and that was the worst he could come up with, so in actuality I felt sorry for myself, but also sorry for Billy for his lack of imagination.

True story. The names have been changed to protect the innocent. Except Billy Strawderman, who was not so innocent. Hope he sees my dust jacket. It's not retouched, either.

(Side Note: I had the pleasure of reconnecting with Billy and his sweet wife at our 25-year high school reunion in New Jersey last summer. I alerted him that I was going to be calling him out about this incident in a public forum in the near future, and we shared quite a chuckle over it. So, yeah, I may actually have him to thank for his comment, for, without it, I wouldn't have had some of the material for this book! Thanks, Billy!)

I started babysitting around this time, and a very slim blonde lady whose kids I watched was apparently unhappy with her figure enough that she had an entire bookshelf laden with diet books with titles like *The Beverly Hills Diet*, which consisted of eating all the fruit you want for days, then bread with butter (or, as I interpreted it, whatever I damn well felt like) on a cheat day once a week. This didn't sound half-bad, plus it was summer so we had tons of fruit in the house.

I went on The Beverly Hills Diet because I wanted to look like I lived in Beverly Hills and figured that this was what everyone in Beverly Hills did to stay skinny, rich and beautiful. Even if you didn't live in Beverly Hills, there was no reason that if you ate like they did in Beverly Hills, you couldn't look and even be just like them!!! I fixed my first Beverly Hills Diet breakfast, which was a cup of pineapple, followed two hours later by about 3 cups of strawberries, followed by a lunch of apples and nectarines, which was followed by several days of severe diarrhea. I never got to the much-anticipated cheat day, but I ended up eating nothing but saltines and white bread for about a week just to regulate myself. It looked like I would never get to Beverly. Hills, that is.

The Poor Man's Anorexia

1981- Age 14. Thank God for my mom's church and their guest speakers!!!! My mom brought me home a book from one of her celebrity seminars – apparently, one of Pat Boone's daughters Cherry Boone had been to hell and back and had written a tell-all book about herself and her family to prove it. My mom, being the darling generous spirit that she is, had been kind enough to grab me an autographed copy of Cherry's book!!!! She couldn't wait to press it into my sticky hands,

9

because I was her oldest daughter, and Cherry was Pat's oldest daughter, and therefore she and Pat and Cherry and I were practically soul-mates, most likely with so much in common!!!!

I know my mom must've not read *Starving For Attention* before gifting me with it, and I'm not even sure she heard Cherry speak, unless Cherry specifically omitted most of the book for her speaking engagement and instead regaled the audience with tales of her dad's white shoes and growing up Christian in Hollywood, et cetera, et cetera.

This was my Bible now. I read it, re-read it, and read it again. It was a how-to instructional on anorexia and bulimia!!! Hallelujah!

After reading the back cover, and seeing that in fact this book was all about how she used to be fat and imperfect then lost a whole bunch of weight and became really fucked up but at least skinny, I flipped right to the picture section, of course. There she was! Normal-weight Cherry, thinner Cherry, skeletal Cherry. Seee??????? It was possible!

I pored over the book, never having heard of such a thing as starving oneself or even better, purging?? I tried both valiantly, and settled into bulimia, which I self-titled the "Poor Man's Anorexia" and which made me feel a tad worse than the entire obsession, since I found myself angry I couldn't be good at anorexia but instead had to cave and actually eat. Still, purging was working great for me, and I whittled away about 35 pounds and landed around 116, where I pretty much stayed from about age 14 to 18.

My methods of purging consisted of the following: eating about 12 chocolatey squares of laxatives; drinking milk-of-magnesia; ingesting several diet pills a day, and eating about 18 aspirin so it would make my stomach hurt and therefore I wouldn't want to eat. When I walked in from school after starving myself all day, I would gorge on sandwiches and stale cookies or whatever was handy and down loads of water, to make throwing up easier. I would throw up several times a day sometimes. I didn't know it then, but it seems that bulimics tend to hover around a safe-looking weight because while they purge, some nutrients and calories stay with the body and therefore the bulimic appears deceptively healthy. I would gage whether I Hated myself or Liked myself based on how long I could go without eating. My record was six days with only 4 2-liter bottles of diet soda and 2 apples. I wished I could've done better....

During this time, I still thought I was fat. People responded to me differently, with more acceptance, but I still felt hideous most of the time. Looking back at photos, I realize I was not at all unattractive, and probably actually was kind of cute.

Meals In A Box

Okay, so fast-forward to about age 20. I had started eating out more, socializing, and packed on several pounds. Eventually I was back where I started. I had a friend who was helping a doctor set up an Opti-Fast clinic, so I tried that. It involved drinking only shakes, and adopting psychotic behavior. No food. I did this for several weeks until the cost and likely the hallucinations caught up to me and I had to stop.

God, I'd be ravenous. I'd picture how food tasted, the act of chewing, the swallowing. I would rent *Willy Wonka and the Chocolate Factory* and fast-forward to all the candy parts, and mimic Violet as she met her blue fate after swiping an Everlasting Gobstopper. I would act out with her the entire scene, tasting the "gravy running down my throat!!" Once I even cut a picture of a turkey dinner out of *Good Housekeeping* magazine and ate it. No lie.

Another friend chatted up something called Nutri-System, wherein you went and plunked down over a thousand dollars and then they let you buy their yellow-boxed food and that's all you ate. You could also have a little fruit and veggies, but that's it. This worked well enough. The tuna was inedible even to a cat. The crackers were so yummy that whenever I bought a box that was to last me a full week, I'd polish off the entire box on the way home from picking up my food. There were meetings to change your eating habits. These consisted mostly of a matronly "counselor" with a flip-chart showing a cartoon of a fat-armed woman (which represented me) with balloons of thoughts like stress, fatigue, self-loathing, etc. flying around her befuddled head. I never paid much attention to these sessions; I was the youngest person there and I felt weird sitting among women my mom's age. I nodded in agreement when asked if I understood why I was the way I was as it pertained to my overeating, and that was that.

I managed to lose about 20 pounds with Nutri-System, and was in a gloriously-great mood for the several months I maintained the weight.

Alas, life changes occurred, I moved away, and my social situation changed drastically. As always, my best friend food was right there for me, and I didn't let her down – I put her up on that pedestal, bestowing all that importance on her as I'd always done, and she repaid me by being there for me, to soothe me, to comfort me, to fatten me up all over again.

My First Rodeo With Cardio

In my early twenties, I managed to lose about thirty pounds doing something extraordinarily risky – I started exercising. (As a funny footnote: Do NOT put this book down now that you've read it and think I've betrayed you, fellow couch potatoans. Ultimately, how I lost my weight and kept it off included pizza, ice cream & chocolate every day if I wanted it. So there. Read on oh ye of little faith).   I took up jogging,

Now, by jogging I mean shuffling my feet more quickly than if I were riding on the back of a turtle who'd overdosed on Thorazine. I am one of those people who, when I'm reading a "how to lose weight" article and I see anywhere on the page the ridiculous suggestions that I "take the stairs instead of the elevator!!!" or "Park farther away from the store!!!", immediately put the magazine down in disgust and make myself a peanut butter & fluff sandwich.   So yeah, my version of exercise was better than what I had been doing, which was usually carrying a silly amount of groceries from the car to the house just so I didn't have to make another twenty-foot trek. I have no idea how I ended up so, well, uninterested in ambulation.

My great-great-great grandfather on my mom's side played for the Brooklyn Dodgers and my mom's whole family were avid sports enthusiasts. Much to the chagrin of my dad, whose family had a more bookish bend and were musicians; still, my dad led our high school marching band for as long as I could remember, and he was always on the move. I myself got out of participating in marching band by pretending that my true calling was piano and therefore Dad would be interrupting my God-given talent if he made me play anything that was portable.

Still, my mom had enrolled me in two years of ballet when I was prepubescent; I recall my teacher vividly, a graying skeletal French woman who chain-smoked while she lorded over her gaggle of 9-year-old students and we had the luxury of breathing in her criticisms and second-hand breath. I also recall that this was when I decided I too would one day devote my life to cigarettes. Which I did from about age 15 to 35. I wistfully look back at all that cigarette money and wonder how many more copies of *Dr. Atkins Diet Revolution* or food scales I could've bought instead.

Ah, I digress. If only ADHD expended calories I'd be able to live in a bakery. Okay, to make my lazy self warm up to such an undertaking, I had to have the clothes and the sneaks. I felt so awkward inside Sports Authority that I immediately wished for a nose & glasses mask to hide beneath. Impossibly fit young people abounded, demanding to know if they could assist.

I saw one lumbering towards me as I turned the corner marked "Running Fashions" (as if). I tried to turn back the way I'd come but my sweater got hooked on a sock rack, which slowed my escape.

"HI!!! CAN I HELP YOU FIND YOUR SIZE???!!!" yelled a butchy saleslady. Bridget, her tag said. I couldn't help but instantly picture her as a Labrador retriever, a friendly barker, if you will. Her tail wagged and her hands were up in a submissive yet helpful manner, as if begging me to let her help. "Here! Bridget! Get the Frisbee! Get the Frisbee, Girl!! Again? You want me to throw it Again??? Oh, Bridget, don't you ever get tired of this GAME?? Nooo, of course you don't, you pretty girl! Good Girl! GOOOOD Girl!"

"Um, yeah, no. no, that's okay. I'm just here…..looking…..here, in your store here."

My largest fear was that someone who clearly had never ingested a morsel of food that was actually edible and not made of tree bark, and who no doubt ate, slept and bathed on a Stairmaster, would catch me trying to buy something exercise-related. I pictured her thoughts sprinting through her short practical haircut, wondering why on earth I, an obvious lard-ass, was here, in her arena. I'm sure she'd seen it all before, and usually in the beginning of January when lard-asses everywhere decided to make a New Year's Resolution to shape up, and then again in May, when all the magazines posed twelve-year old Brazilian supermodels on their covers reminding us that this was the month we had to try on bathing suits so we better hurry it up and join a gym. Note: by "join a gym" I of course mean giving a gym your bank account number so that they can feel free to direct-debit your bank account $49.99 a month for the rest of your life, and then do the same to your heirs and your heirs' heirs. You must thereby agree to only go to this gym a maximum of 40 days, and then be distracted, then guilt-ridden, ashamed, and never set foot there again. I imagine in 3009, scientists will unearth evidence of this phenomenon and laugh their asses off.

I started walking slowly away from Bridget, backwards, slowly, in case she turned Cujo. She allowed my retreat with a shoulder shrug and trotted away to find someone who knew what they wanted and where they were going.

I fumbled through some sale racks, because I knew myself well enough by now – spending hundreds of dollars on running clothes does not make one want to run. I selected several long pants (medium, which since what I had in girth I lacked in height, and I'd end up having to turn the waistband down so I could walk), long-sleeved dri-weave tops (large), and a few jogging bras (large). On to the shoes, I picked some that I'd heard of that looked cute and didn't have either pink or purple on them.

My eyes wandered over the videotape racks, saw blonde grinning forty-somethings with twenty-year old bodies folded nearly in half. Over the big balls and little balls and resistance bands. I pictured myself using all of these things, then I quickly pictured myself falling off the ball and smashing my head and trying to explain how that happened and decided to stick to employing just my own body for now.

At this time, I was in a tremendously unequal long-term relationship with a much older man, who apparently had been put on this earth to control me. I allowed this for years, but as our tenure drew to a close, I found I used this as an impetus to running. The more trapped I felt, the more I was able to get up each day and run. Sort of a self-imposed punishment for staying where I should not.

I would be out the door while the moon was still up, so no one would see me jiggling and puffing up the street. I wore my headphones and carried my little Walkman, and listened to Michael Jackson, Cake, Dire Straits, a collection of 70's stuff. "You're no good! You're no good! You're no good, baby you're no goooooood!" Linda Ronstadt reminded me that I could in fact channel my inability to level the playing field with my beau into beating myself into an exercise routine that I stuck with for about two years.

Life Changes...Which Changed My Life

Enter the breakup. I wasn't at an ideal weight, but I had gotten down to a range where I felt I could accept invitations to public gatherings and find something to wear to them in my own closet. I had jeans I didn't need to be a contortionist to don and that didn't cause lack of lower extremity blood-flow.

Sure, I might have been able to reach my goal weight, but honestly, when you lose some weight, sycophants come out of the woodwork. See, most people want to lose weight and try valiantly nearly every day of their lives. I know because I've done it and know countless others just like me. Rarely do people succeed, and so when they do, there are plenty of compliments offered up to them.

"Where's the rest of you!!! What have you done!!! You look so different!" Blah blah blah. The problem is, most of us believe our own ink at that stage of loss and never go the distance. Any weight loss is an accomplishment, but truth be told, there was no reason for me to stop exercising. I wasn't "done" yet, and exercise, as our logical mind knows, isn't something we do for a while to lose weight or improve our health, only to abandon it once we start fitting into our skinny jeans.

However, this is what I did, and after the breakup, I met a cute younger guy whom I eventually married. By this time, I was up several pounds but he didn't seem to mind and I didn't seem to notice in time to do anything about it. Why is it that happiness in a new relationship equals eating whatever we want and throwing our routine to the wind? Is it that self-disappointment spurs us to make changes? Is it that we feel we've found someone who likes us for who we are not what we look like, again, an invalid argument, but one that allows us to have our cake and eat it, too? My younger sister, a newlywed, calls it the Newlywed Nineteen.

By this point, I was in my mid-thirties. I weighed about 35 or 40 pounds more than what I wanted to, and I was disgusted with myself most of the time. My husband would advise us of invitations to go boating, beaching, etc. and I would always come up with excuses for why I couldn't go but he was welcome to. He sometimes went, and sometimes didn't, but I'm sure he was always perplexed as to why I never wanted to go anywhere.

We were also trying to conceive, which gave me full license to eat whatever I wanted. Um, yeah, no, pregnancy might lull you into thinking you can eat the entire refrigerator contents whenever you damn well please, but conceiving? Not so much. No one ever tells you this, but trying to conceive is not picking out paint swatches in a sunlit nursery while your husband lovingly cradles your Baby Bump. It's about eating crap, feeling like crap, peeing on sticks, anxiety, desperation, and frustration. I consoled myself with food.

In October 2003, after suffering seven miscarriages, work with fertility doctors (it should be noted that both of my babies were conceived naturally after fertility attempts failed), my husband and I finally conceived a child. His name was Hunter. I carried him for twenty-eight weeks, at which time I went into premature labor after a placental abruption. He and I were both touch and go. When he was born, he was in the NICU. I held him and sang to him every day, pumped breast milk for the nurses to feed him, and looked forward with boundless nervous excitement to the day we'd bring him home to his much-planned nursery. But our love was not enough to keep him here.

After one short month, he passed away due to a medical error, leaving a void I could never hope to describe. It's years later, and I have two more beautiful children, but not a day passes when I don't miss Hunter or feel his presence in my heart, or feel the loss of what might have been, what is missing. He's not here with me, but he's not gone, either. He's my firstborn, my third child I love and know, yet don't get to be with, and that leaves a grief that just stays with you, and it affects all that you do and why you do it. You evaluate your two lives - the one you lived up to that point of loss, and the life you attempt to construct after.

Which brings me to how I finally got my ass in gear and why you're reading my book.

Life is short. We all know it, and it's a cliché. However, after years of wishing your child here, then you're blessed with his birth, and then in a month he's just gone, you need to somehow make sense of it. But that's impossible, because bad things happen to good people every day. I pulled strength that I had no business having out of my depths and plunged into a journey of making every day of my own life count and live happily, since Hunter was denied the opportunity. I live for him. I'm living for two.

CHAPTER TWO
Why Diets Fail (And We All Know They Do)

Okay, ready for this: It's the calories, stupid. Really! Here's how:

A pound = 3,500 calories. There are seven days in a week, although if you have kids, it seems like 14, especially in summer.

$3,500 \div 7 = 500$

Therefore, you need to create a 500-calorie deficit every day in order to lose about a pound a week.

What's funny is that whether we realize it or not, *every diet out there involves calorie reduction*, it's just usually not presented as such. Think about it: Weight Watchers has its food plan, which consists of consuming between 1,100 and 1,500 calories per day. Atkins, by the time you've been strict for about a week or so, also ends up being a calorie-reduced plan, because how many blocks of cheese and sticks of butter can you really eat without eventually settling down and eating lean proteins which are less calorie-dense than say, cheese? South Beach Diet, Nutri-System, Jenny Craig, The Cookie Diet, The Zone, the list goes on & on. So after I came to this realization, I started delving into my dieting history to see what had ever worked and what had never worked.

Why had I historically "fallen off" my diet?

Because "diets" are impractical. I would be forced to change my eating habits drastically by not eating my favorite foods like pizza, ice cream, chips, chocolate, and booze. Any diet that told me I had to eat lean portions of fish and salad and yet deprived me of my glass of wine and a sundae at the end of the day made me incredibly angry after about three days, leading soon to over-indulging, almost in a panic. *"I love you Chardonnay, I'm so sorry I strayed! I'll never leave you again!"*

What had worked in the past? Well, for me, I do like Jenny Craig because I could have my yummy foods and still lose weight. However, for me, there had always been two downfalls with this plan: one, the food was really expensive for my budget, usually about $100 to $130 a week for me to buy the foods I needed to stick to it; and two, there was no room for error. Meaning, if I were invited to lunch or for an after-work drink, I was technically "off" and therefore would have extra food at the end of the week. My counselors were always pretty nice about this, but they raised eyebrows and implored me to stick to the plan despite it interfering with me wanting to socialize.

I feel like unless you live in a bubble, having the luxury of never going out, never being confronted with a candy dish or a surprise party, or a holiday, or your kids simply wanting you to have bites of something they're enjoying, then you need an approach that is not all-or-nothing.

The all-or-nothing approach doesn't work. It's too radical, and life is not black and white; it's gray. In order to lose more than a few pounds, you will need to eat to lose for weeks and maybe months. So, in order for that to happen, you need to learn substitutes for your favorite foods, you need to learn how to eat one or two of something that you know will slow your weekly loss, and you need to get your head out of the guilt.

For example, if you have one cookie, you might say to yourself, "Well, I blew it. I will now eat the entire sleeve and then continue to eat crazy until the following Monday when I will start my diet over." My entire dieting career was lived with this mindset, and it took something profound for me to really discover this. A bobble here and there, even many throughout the week, if kept in check, does NOT mean you won't lose weight!!! It's actually necessary for you to have bobbles, because this is your new life, your new way of eating, rather than eating one way while you're losing, then eating another way once you've arrived and now need to maintain!!!

If you run a red light and get a ticket, does that mean you should then continue breaking every traffic law you can for the rest of the day? One cookie, or even two, usually is only about 75 to 150 calories of damage. All that means is that later in the day, instead of having a low-fat frozen yogurt ice cream cone, you could instead choose to have a 60-calorie pudding with a squirt of whipped cream and some fruit. You will make up that 150-calorie bobble earlier in the day by making this choice, and you will STILL be having TWO treats – one treat is the dessert, and the other treat is that the scale will continue moving downward!!! Everybody wins!! You need to hone this new perspective, so treat bobbles not as major screw-ups, but as learning opportunities. Cut yourself slack; chances are you've been doing the "eating right / bobble / guilt / overeat rest of week / start diet again

Monday" cycle forever, so undoing this mindset doesn't happen overnight but it WILL happen.

Equally important is to know that, much like waiting until you can afford to have kids, there will never be a perfect time to diet. This is why DIETS DON'T WORK. They have a definite beginning and end. They begin sincerely with breakfast, usually on a Monday and by Wednesday, after torturing yourself with dry tuna, celery, lack of carbohydrates, watery soups and Jell-o, black coffee, etc. you are confronted with the following scenario:

"It's Mel's birthday!!! Ya know, Mel....from accounting! There's cake in the conference room!!!! Come!" "Um, no, I have to finish up this file..." "NOOOO! It's an order! Let's go!"

And so it goes. Or...

"A bunch of us are meeting for happy hour at that martini place, that guy I've been telling you about will be there..."

Or...

"Mrs. Miller, we're having a bake sale Friday so could you make brownies or chocolate chip cookies?"

Real life is where we live, and the best laid plans of mice & men are no match for a classic diet. Even if you could overcome these situational eating pratfalls, give you one bad day, an overdue bill, angry words with a spouse, and before you know it you're elbow-deep in pie. What's funny is that food's used universally as a comfort, when in actuality once we stop the feeding frenzy and look back at what we've done, we are left feeling anything but comfort. Instead, feelings of shame, guilt, hopelessness, and self-hatred abound. Self-soothing with

24

food is most likely infantile- but we all do it. This book contains fabulous substitutes- from my personal experience and those of my success clients- which are very low in calorie but are wonderfully satisfying.

You will see how people who seem not to watch their weight stay the same size year after year – they eat when they're hungry, stop before they're full, and give themselves permission to have yummies but don't act as if that's the last chance they'll ever get face-time with a treat. If you want another brownie, for example, don't freak out and eat four; just say calmly to yourself, "Hey, I could eat that tomorrow if I want another one. I don't have to act like I'll never have another brownie again for a year because of my 'diet,' so I'll stop with this one, and then tomorrow will come and I'll decide then if I really want to eat it." Research has shown time and time again that eating a small amount of something we crave usually satisfies our craving, so we can stop obsessing about it and move forward with our weight loss!

CHAPTER THREE
Why My Plan Works (I Promise!)

So back to the 500-calorie deficit issue:

What can 500 calories look like? Let's look at typical 500 calorie combinations:

-A bakery bagel with cream cheese

-2 doughnut-shop doughnuts

-A large piece of fried chicken

-A typical cheeseburger with condiments

-A typical deli sandwich (meat, cheese and mayo)

-A few tablespoons of creamy salad dressing

-A tuna salad sandwich

-A small chicken Caesar salad

-A fast-food single cheeseburger and small fries

-A large baked potato with butter & sour cream

-A slice of ice cream cake

-A slice of pie

-Two fried eggs, two slices of bacon and toast

Okay. **So, what I did (and what you'll do too) was find a way to cut calories here and there and replace foods with other foods that were higher-volume** (think getting more bang for your buck, or more food for the calories).

For example, say I crave potato chips (if you don't, I'm not your friend anymore). I could crack open a big bag and start digging in, feeling remorse and self-loathing with each delicious bite. Or I could crack open a smaller bag and dig in. Either way, if you look at the calories per serving of even a small bag, it's usually 2 servings in there and the calories are usually at least 250 per serving. If what my mouth and hands need are salt and something to reach into a bag repeatedly for, then why can't I try a 100-calorie bag of potato chips? Or tortilla chips, or cheese puffs? Eaten slowly and guilt-freely.

Better yet, if I must have salt and crunch, maybe I don't need it to be chips. Sure, once in a while it MUST be chips, but I found a satisfying alternative for the majority of my snacking. Since chips are high in the fat/salt/crunch area but not the best nutritional choice, then why not try a 100-calorie bag of butter flavored popcorn? Or kettle corn? Making sure the bag is in fact a 100-calorie bag and not 100 calories per serving is key. You'll be reading labels from now on, just to start familiarizing yourself with calories – how many calories are in a serving. For instance, I'm no stranger to reaching into a jar of nuts and fishing through the big fat yucky Brazil nuts (which my dad and maybe 2 other people like) for the pecans. However, the one time I actually bothered to look at the nutritional label of my giant jar o' nuts from the price-club warehouse, I snatched my salt-covered fingers back out as if the jar was filled with tarantulas when I realized that a serving of the nuts consisted of about 2 tablespoons of nuts and was about 200 calories. Okay. Do it with me: go get a tablespoon out of your drawer and look at it. Now measure out some nuts into it. No cheating, no overage, no air rights. See how many nuts that is? Or isn't??

So, the choice will be yours my friend: Can you have nuts? Sure, of course. And actually, they are a great choice nutritionally-speaking – they contain vitamins and fiber, and healthy fats. However, please make sure that you can stop when you need to. A great way to do this would be to put a serving in a small baggie and put the jar back in the cabinet where it's out of sight and enjoy your baggie of nuts as you walk away from the kitchen.

Which brings me to another big huge adjustment I made when I started my weight loss journey: **Start being honest with yourself**. If you're bothering to do this plan, then that means you are really, really, really sick of dieting and you'd love, love, love to get this weight off as quickly as is safely possible. I am showing you how a regular person broke a lifetime of dieting and lost all my weight and then some, and have kept it off. So why play with it? Why pretend you didn't just lick that spoon when you made your kids PB & J sandwich? That could've been 50 calories… calories you might rather have at the day's end in low-fat frozen yogurt! Or if you're fudging on goldfish-shaped crackers, and rather than count them out or measure out a ¼ cup like the serving size says, and you're just loosey-goosey with it, you only have yourself to blame for slowing your weight loss. Be Honest With Yourself. And then congratulate yourself with every good thing you do, every wiser choice you make.

This next part is I think the most important part of this plan, and it was my turning point: **When you eat something you weren't planning on, you must forgive yourself**. You must forgive yourself, register whether it was worth it (and sometimes it will be – a special piece of cake perhaps, or a yummy cheese at a party that you'll never see again). Register how you feel about it – when I was in my loss phase, I would even go as far as to write in my food journal how I felt afterward. This is key in making this not another diet, but a way of eating to get thin and then keeping the weight off.

Remember to ask yourself, "What would I be eating if I weren't eating this (on-plan) food? If I weren't eating to lose weight, I'd be having, say a peanut butter & jelly sandwich…" Well, you CAN HAVE THAT! I did. I'd make a lower-calorie peanut butter & sugar-free grape jelly on very thin sliced whole wheat bread – I would use three slices of bread (110 calories for 3 slices), a tablespoon of peanut butter for the bread (about 70-90 calories) and 2 tsp sugar-free jelly (about 20 calories). So, you see, for about a third or less of the calories you'd get from a traditional PB&J sandwich, you have the EXACT same flavor but with zero guilt - and the scale needle goes down.

Sometimes I even like the weird combo of potato chips inside my sandwich (don't ask – my family's from Kentucky and that should be enough information), so I'd crack open a 100-calorie pack of kettle-cooked potato chips and put half the package inside my sandwiches and save the other half for a rainy day. If I were NOT trying to lose weight, this is EXACTLY what I'd be craving and caving in to – it doesn't have to be that way! There are substitutions for everything you could crave, and I have a whole section in this book with substitutions for you to try.

Remember, this is NOT a diet; it's a new approach to food, a new way of exploring how you eat, why you eat, when and where.

I want the years of yo-yo dieting to be *history*. My plan is not about being "on" or "off" a diet; diets have a beginning and an end which is why they don't work long-term and it's hard to keep the weight off after they're "over." You will learn new habits that encompass eating when you're hungry and seeing food as a part of your day, but your day will no longer revolve around it! You'll eat when you're physically hungry, stop before you feel stuffed, and you will no longer use food as a tasteless crutch. Food will become something to enjoy, a pleasure, a comfort, a social enjoyment, *but without the guilt! You will be liberated at last from food guilt!!*

This plan is about enjoying *all* foods and beverages in moderation. It's about having some days where you eat more calories than average and making it up to yourself and keeping on course by having a little less other days, in essence to balance out your daily intake, so that you can continue to lose weight until you reach your goal, and then maintain it, *forever breaking the cycle of dieting. It's about being in control.*

A "Black and White", "All or Nothing" approach absolutely does not work with eating. It can work with alcohol, smoking, relationships, and pretty much everything else, except eating. You cannot stop eating altogether. It's also pretty difficult and, frankly, depressing, to forever rule out any specific food group, such as carbohydrates. It would be very sad to have to forever deny yourself dessert, or a favorite holiday treat. *It's incredibly unrealistic.* This plan works and others do not because this plan is not extreme, it doesn't ask you to radically alter how you normally eat, just the portion sizes, and it eliminates the most unhealthy foods by substituting them for wiser yet equally satisfying alternatives. Instead of wishing you were "done" with your diet so you can "hurry up and have ," you will already be enjoying it but in healthier doses that enable you to reach your goal and not feel guilty on the journey!

Knowing you can still have the foods you love (or a lower-calorie variation) every single day and still lose weight will enable you to have a completely different mindset this time!

You can do this. Let me help you reclaim yourself.

I have been on your journey and know you will succeed! You have a right to be the person you are. Own it.

CHAPTER FOUR

Tips & Tricks: On Your Way to Your Goal

I've learned a few tips and tricks along the way that have helped me. Hopefully some of them will be useful to you as well.

Try not to drink your calories. If you are used to drinking juice and soda, you will be happily surprised when you see how cutting these out will help you create your calorie deficit right away. If you must drink juice, I suggest cutting it with water and/or club soda and working it out of your diet. Fruit is a healthier alternative to juice and will be more filling.

Hydrate constantly. If you don't already carry a water bottle everywhere with you, start. Buy a cool one (no pun intended). Keep it filled with ice water, sugar-free drink mix, or iced tea. I like cold-brewed iced tea mixed with sugar-free lemonade in a giant cup of ice and a little water. I drink it all day; it keeps my mouth busy and my body properly hydrated.

Green tea is a wonderful twist on tea (hot or cold) and is shown to reduce belly bloat and aid digestion, and it's also rich in antioxidants. Coffee is permissible; try not to add much cream but a little is ok. Remember to count cream/creamers in your calorie plan for the day. Artificial sweeteners can be used sparingly.

Drinking makes us feel full. Additionally, sometimes we feel hungry when we are in fact thirsty. Get in the habit of bringing water or a water bottle with acceptable fluid with you everywhere you go!

Regarding diet soda: if you have a sweet tooth, there are several delicious diet sodas available now, such as diet orange cream, diet root beer, and diet cream soda. Again, try to limit to one a day, but if you're used to many, cut down gradually until you're at one a day or one every now and then. You can also make low-calorie root beer floats with this soda and low-fat frozen vanilla yogurt or light whipped topping, or an orange Creamsicle-tasting drink with the diet orange soda & whipped topping. Use your imagination!

An alternative to any meal or snack is juicing. If you have a juicer, congrats! You are the proud owner of a $300 kitchen gadget that collects more dust than your stair-stepper. Just kidding- sort of! If you don't have one, do what I do: pre-made juices or smoothies. Just choose ones that are low in calories (fewer than 150/serving- read label to make sure what a serving size is). Drink it & you've eaten lots of fruit & veggies. Plus, you'll get that smug feeling that tri-athletes probably get when they're downing something that looks like a prop from *The Exorcist*.

Bars are a convenient and nutritious way to make sure you're never without something to put in your mouth. I prefer kid-sized bars (usually 140 calories vs. 200+ for regular bars) and my kids dig them, too. Some brands and varieties have more calories than others, so read labels.

Keep one stashed somewhere (like your purse, glove compartment, desk drawer, etc.) at all times so if you're experiencing a craving and before you feel starved, you can reach for one to take the edge off.

With proper planning (and aren't you worth it?), there is never a good reason to give fast-food joints any more of your money because you're famished. I don't always eat the bars in lieu of fresh food, but if I'm in a rush and don't have fruit or cheeses or veggies on hand to grab, then I know I'm covered. *The trick is to pre-plan and always have alternatives on hand, plus a safety net, so you don't fall prey to a vending machine or fast food.*

For instance, pick two days a week (Sunday /Wed?) for chopping/bagging/ freezing sauces, fruits, crackers, et cetera, putting together snacks to grab in an instant.

And it's really, really important to pack a cooler or lunchbox for yourself when you're on the road - that way you have no excuse to NOT have proper foods in the car! Many people, moms in particular, spend tons of time in their car. If you're starving, it's too tempting to pull up to a fast-food window or convenience store. You love their kids enough to pack THEM a lunch - love yourself enough. One nutritionist speaks of this as arming yourself for battle - against all the neon fast-food signs you pass along the road.

Good items to include would be fruit, yogurt & plastic spoon, bottled water, a small bag of nuts, cheese sticks, deli roll-ups, and any kind of reduced-fat wheat crackers. I do this every day. I'm in my car all the time, and it helps- I promise you!

Another trick – for a low-calorie snack, try having a bowl of blueberries or strawberries with a couple tablespoons of crunchy cereal sprinkled on top and a little skim milk.

Experiment with salads. Add as much strong flavor, color and crunch as possible to any salad so that your mouth, taste buds and brain have all registered that you have in fact eaten a lot!

Portions are really important. Portions = calories.

Protein: Should be 2-3 oz. per serving. A good guideline is to use your fingers from top of palm to fingertips….or you can use a 3 oz. can of tuna as your guide. Another trick I use is that when I'm getting lunch meat, I ask the deli person to weigh 3 oz. of meat, then put paper, then another 3 oz., then put paper, etc. They never mind doing it, and it gives you exactly what you need portion-wise, plus it allows to you eventually eyeball the amount without having to buy a food scale!

Carbs: Check your serving sizes for calories – since I'm a grazer, I tend to like reduced-fat crackers, but really any whole-grain or whole wheat cracker will suffice. Just be sure to check your serving sizes & calories – most crackers like these are around 16 crackers for 130 calories – but this can vary.

Breads: Shoot for breads / English muffins / pita – that give you the most bang for your calorie buck. For example – can you have a raisin English Muffin? Sure you can! But know that they are about 140 calories vs. 100 for a light whole grain variety…you can have either, or you might see that you'd rather spend that 40 extra calories somewhere else later in the day (½ glass of wine, bank the 40 towards a 100 calorie dessert, etc.) – the choice is yours. But if you want to go for a higher-calorie version – know that you CAN, but write down the calories so you're not fooling yourself. ☺

Condiments: I found that I really liked fitting into a bathing suit much more than I liked mayonnaise! I got used to using the little triangles of light cheese (35 calories per wedge) on my sandwiches or roll-ups instead. Or mustard – check calories, but most are between 5 and 20 per tsp. Another GREAT substitute for me were the new spray-on butter substitutes – I am a big butter / margarine fan – but the calories just weren't worth it. Occasionally, sure, but for most days, not worth the calories to moisten bread!!! Most varieties are around 0-5 calories a spray.

Likewise with salad dressing – I am a huge blue-cheese dressing girl, but even the low-calorie versions are about 100 calories per serving. I cut calories by using a spray-on variety (at 1 calorie per spray!) and, when I had to, I would get fresh blue-cheese crumbles and use a teaspoon of those on my salad with the spray-on dressing! The real blue cheese dressing has about 30-50 calories per teaspoon – another reduction of calories that I never even noticed I was giving up. So you can see that just by making, for example, the margarine change-up and the salad dressing change-up, I saved over 100 calories without even trying!!

This plan is, again, all about substitutions, food modification, and portion control, NOT about deprivation!!!!! Deprivation for me (and most people) = not being able to stick to a traditional "diet" long enough to lose weight!!!!!

Regarding veggies & fruit – I don't even ask my clients to write down their veggie consumption – I'm a firm believer that you cannot go wrong eating large amounts of fresh (or frozen) veggies (avoiding potatoes, kidney beans & garbanzo beans – you can still have them, but you need to count their calories in your log). The great thing I learned about veggies, too, is that because they are SO LOW in calories and so high in nutritional value & hunger satisfaction, they can and should be eaten in abundance. Roast them with a drizzle of olive oil (or olive oil cooking spray), a sprinkle of seasoning (garlic powder, etc.) and a sprinkle of cheese!! Two of my favorite veggie dishes are just steaming up a big bowl of fresh green beans (throw them in a bowl with a little water & nuke for about 3 minutes); then I put cracked black pepper on them and toss in about a tsp. of freshly-grated good Parmesan cheese – I still eat these all the time! I even carry a baggie of them, cold, in my purse!!! Very very filling and about 40 calories max!!!

Re: Fruit – you should include them in your calorie log, but bear in mind that I have the same attitude about them that I do about veggies – most have negligible calories if you factor in how great they are for you, and how filling – plus, they're pretty and fun to eat (fresh or frozen). They have high water content too so they make your skin look wonderful!!! All berries are great choices, as are apples. Melon, also. I say, when it comes to fruit & veggies, go for it! No one ever gained weight by eating too many fruits & veggies ☺ Also a great habit to pass onto our kiddos….

If you're busy (who isn't), I also became a big fan of buying trays of fresh fruits & veggies…sure, they're a little more expensive, but hey – it looks like company's coming over! Plus, how many times have you let heads of broccoli and bags of apples rot in your "crisper"? That's really a waste of money – the trays will get eaten, I promise!

As soon as I bring a veggie tray home, I immediately take out the dressing dip and toss it – instead, I get 100-calorie fat-free plain yogurt, and mix in about a ¼ packet of onion or veggie soup mix and use that as a dip. I get the exact same satisfaction as I would from the dip or dressing that comes with the tray, without hating myself in the morning!!!

Get creative with fruits and vegetables. Try freezing fresh-cut fruit, such as peaches, all berries, mandarin oranges, and grapes. They take longer to eat and have a satisfying texture…you can also add frozen fruit to yogurt and frozen yogurt for a sweet healthy treat!

Yogurt is great to have on hand at all times. Keep the calorie count between 100 and 140. There are lots of great flavors out there, even ones that taste like dessert. Read your labels, as some brands make "light" and also sugar-free and reduced calorie. You could end up with 240 calorie ones if you aren't careful, so be sure to read, and be sure it's 1 serving per package!

Experiment with desserts – you can take a day where you have both frozen yogurt and 100-calorie pack of cookies allowed, and combine them to make "blend-ins" which are smooth, crunchy, and sweet all at the same time. You'll know what you're in the mood for, and it will probably change from day to day.

Also handy and tasty are the new 60-calorie puddings, especially the chocolate and banana-chocolate parfait flavors. You can even top with whipped light cream! Excellent for curbing a sweet tooth. I also recently found chocolate-covered frozen bananas at 140 calories each – so yummy.

Lastly, regarding the inevitable junk food:

Get familiar with all the 100-calorie snack packs out there – if you're craving cheese puffs or cookies, I say – have it! Rather than making yourself feel deprived because you're dying for something you think you cannot have – go ahead & have it – but have a controlled portion of it, so you're not doing damage to your calorie count for the day.

If you don't have 100-calorie snack packs, have one or two or the thing you're craving – for example, I LOVE chocolate-covered mint cookies – before losing weight, I would have one, then say "oh, I blew it – now I might as well eat the whole sleeve and start my diet over tomorrow." Can you see how ridiculous that looks on paper??? One or two cookies generally have 70-140 calories! Go ahead and indulge when you need to, and get rid of the mindset that says "I might as well eat them all and start over again tomorrow" – that does not work!!! If you have something considered "junk", just include it in your calorie log, taste them, enjoy them, and then say "hey, if I want, I can have more tomorrow". This is a never say "I can't have that" approach – it's about MODERATION AND SUBSTITUTION, and including much more nutritious foods and less of the junk! I firmly believe that it's this mindset that separates those who maintain a normal weight throughout their lives from those of us who tend to get on a diet roller coaster.

It's also important to eat every two to three hours. Blood sugar needs to be stable in order for you to not get headaches, feel grouchy, and feel true hunger. Plus, when you're throwing a log on the fire that is your metabolism every two hours or so, you're burning more efficiently. Pre-planning with handy, yummy portable foods will be the key to staving off hunger which can lead to screw-ups.

Also, presentation is important. Try not to eat standing over the sink out of a container whenever possible. Try putting your food on really elegant plates, having a pretty table setting, using nice glassware, etc. *Be nice to yourself!*

If you're feeding your kids, resist the urge to eat their leftovers. Really, is that spoonful of cold mac 'n cheese or that last rubbery chicken nugget worth the calories? The best thing to do is clean up their plates and immediately scrape them into the garbage or into the sink disposal. That way you won't even be tempted.

It's a work in progress, and it's a re-thinking of how we normally approach "dieting" – you WILL lose all the weight you want to lose doing this plan, and better yet, you'll maintain it easily because you'll have implemented sound eating habits – plus, you'll be rocking your new figure, which is an obvious incentive to stay in control!!!!

IF I CAN DO THIS, SO CAN YOU! ☺

CHAPTER FIVE

Shopping List: Don't Leave Home Without It

BREAD / CRACKERS / CEREAL – NO WHITE !	DAIRY
□ Pita pockets, halved, whole wheat	□ Fat-free half & half
□ 100-calorie whole grain English Muffins	□ Skim milk
□ Very thin-sliced wheat bread (or any non-white bread that's 30-50 cal/sl)	□ Low- or non-fat cottage cheese in single-serve packs
□ Low-fat wheat crackers	□ Low-fat cheese sticks (mozzarella, cheddar, etc. 80-100 cals each)
□ Multigrain crackers	□ Greek yogurt (blueberry, vanilla, plain) 100-120 cals ea.
□ Crisp breads	□ Non-fat or light yogurt, up to 120 cals ea.
□ Melba Rounds/ Toast	□ Egg whites / eggs
□ Ice cream cones (cake) – 20 cals	□ Light cheese – wedges / cubes
□ Oatmeal (steel-cut)	□ Shredded Parm & Romano cheeses
□ Grits	□ Spray-on Butter substitute – 0-5 cals / serving
□ 100-Calorie snack packs (cookies, pretzels, chips)	□ Low-fat cream cheese
□ Whole-grain cereal (3/4 – 1 cu. at appx. 90-130 cals)	□ Non-fat sour cream
	□ Whipped cream (reg/light/choc)

ADDITIONAL FROZEN FOODS	VEGETABLES
☐ Veggie sausage links	☐ Green beans (fresh)
☐ Turkey sausage links	☐ Asparagus (fresh)
☐ Any diet frozen entrees (less than 300 cal/serving)	☐ Zucchini
☐ Low-fat frozen yogurt	☐ Onions / Garlic
☐ No-sugar-added fudge bars	☐ Peppers
☐ 10-cal frozen bars	☐ Sweet potato
☐ Mini ice cream cones or sandwiches	☐ Artichoke hearts (in water)
☐ Any frozen diet dessert btw. 10 & 150 cals	☐ Hearts of palm (in water)
☐ Light whipped topping – reg/choc/strawberry	☐ Tomatoes
FRUIT	☐ Sundried tomatoes
☐ Apples	☐ Baby carrots
☐ Dark Grapes	☐ Leaf spinach
☐ Citrus	☐ Salad (bagged is easiest)
☐ Plums, Peaches, Nectarines	☐ Cucumbers
☐ Melon (all kinds)	☐ Arugula
☐ Blueberries, strawberries	☐ Cilantro

MEAT / POULTRY / SEAFOOD	MISCELLANEOUS
□ Ground turkey, beef - fresh or frozen	□ 0-calorie chocolate sauce and/or dip
□ Veggie burgers	□ Marshmallow dip
□ Chicken breast	□ Salad dressing – any spray-on kind that's 1 cal / spray
□ Shrimp	□ Diet hot chocolate (40 cals / packet or less)
□ Salmon or other fish filets	□ 60-cal soup packets
□ Sushi (avoid mayo-added kind, avoid white rice)	□ Any soup that's 100 cals or less per serving
□ Canned white tuna & chicken (in water)	□ Mustard
□ Deli sliced chicken, turkey, etc. (the leaner the better)	□ Pickles
	□ Capers
	□ 10-cal gelatin dessert
	□ 60-cal pudding (esp. Banana Fudge)
	□ Any nutritional bar under 150 cal.
	□ Sugar-free drink mixes
	□ Diet soda/ sparkling water

CHAPTER SIX: Fixed Menu Plan

You know who you are. You're organized, like to know what the day brings, you plan ahead. If you feel more comfortable on a fixed menu, then here's a 28-day one for you. Follow it for a month and you will see some FANTASTIC results!

Menu: Week 1

Day One	Day Two	Day Three	Day Four
BREAKFAST Lowfat Breakfast Burrito Coffee / Tea w/creamer	**BREAKFAST** ½ Pita pocket toasted w/ spray-on butter 2 veggie or turkey sausages Coffee / Tea w/creamer	**BREAKFAST** 100 cal. English muffin w/ spray butter 1 veggie or turkey sausage Coffee / Tea w/creamer	**BREAKFAST** 3 egg whites, fresh spinach & 1 tbsp shredded cheese 2 slices v. thin wheat bread w/ spray butter Coffee / Tea w/creamer
SNACK Small apple Light cheese (1 wedge or 5 cubes)	**SNACK** Light cheese (1 wedge or 5 cubes) Snack bag of baby carrots ½ nutritional bar	**SNACK** ½ pita pocket w/few slivers sundried tomato, arugula, 2 slices deli chicken, spray 1-cal. Drsg	**SNACK** ½ nutritional bar ½ cup berries
LUNCH Diet frozen entree Huge salad with free veggies & 1-calorie drsg	**LUNCH** Huge salad w/1 can 100-cal. tuna or chicken &1-cal drsg 16 wheat crackers	**LUNCH** Leftover salmon over huge salad w/1-cal drsg Small handful walnuts or almonds	**LUNCH** Diet frozen entree Huge salad w/free vegs & 1-cal drsg
SNACK Nutritional bar **SNACK #2** (*if you eat dinner late*) 2 deli meat roll-ups made with 1-cal. drsg, hearts of palm, sun dried tomatoes Small Nectarine	**SNACK** Antipasto with grilled peppers, marinated artichoke hearts, lunch meat, sprinkle fresh grated parm & romano **SNACK #2** (*if you eat dinner late*) One bag 100-cal. snack ½ apple	**SNACK** Nutritional Bar **SNACK #2** (*if you eat dinner late*) 1 cup mixed berries w/ lowfat whipped topping	**SNACK** 2 deli roll-ups 2 dill pickle spears **SNACK #2** (*if you eat dinner late*) 1 100-cal yogurt Small nectarine or plum
DINNER 1 or 2 bags 100-cal Microwave popcorn ½ cup dark grapes **Or** 1 cup whole grain cereal w/skim milk 1 fruit **DESSERT** 1 small cone w/appx 2 scoops low-fat frozen yogurt ("fro-yo")	**DINNER** Grilled salmon w/ spinach, tomato& capers 1 cup green beans w/ spray butter & sprinkle parm 1 gl wine or 1 vodka/soda **DESSERT** ¼ cup frozen dark chocolate pieces ½ cup fro-yo	**DINNER** 1 or 2 bags 100-cal Microwave popcorn **Or** 1 cup whole grain cereal w/skim milk 1 fruit **DESSERT** small cone w/ appx 2 scoops fro-yo	**DINNER** Grilled Shrimp Roasted asparagus Salad w/arugula, few walnuts and ½ pear 1 gl wine or vod/soda **DESSERT** Frozen bar (100 cals or less)

Menu: Week 1

Day Five	Day Six	Day Seven
BREAKFAST ½ Pita toasted w/spray butter 2 veggie or turkey sausages Coffee/Tea w/creamer	**BREAKFAST** Lowfat Breakfast Burrito Coffee / Tea w/creamer	**BREAKFAST** 3 egg whites w/Cooking spray, fresh spinach, tomato & 1 tbsp shredded cheese 100-cal. Eng. muffin w/ spray butter Coffee /Tea w/creamer
SNACK Snack bag of baby carrots 5 cubes Light cheese ½ Nutritional Bar	**SNACK** 1 100-calorie yogurt w/sprinkle crunchy cereal	**SNACK** 1 100-calorie yogurt w/ ½ small apple
LUNCH Huge salad w/leftover grilled shrimp &1-cal drsg 1 Crisp bread	**LUNCH** Diet frozen entree Huge salad w/1-cal drsg	**LUNCH** Diet frozen entree Huge salad w/1-cal drsg
SNACK Antipasto with grilled peppers, marinated artichoke hearts, lunch meat, sprinkle fresh grated parm & romano ½ small apple **SNACK #2** *(if you eat dinner late)* 1 100-calorie yogurt	**SNACK** ½ Nutritional Bar **SNACK #2** *(if you eat dinner late)* 1 cup mixed berries w/ lowfat whipped topping Light cheese (5 cubes or 1 wedge)	**SNACK** 1 cup honey nut circles cereal (in baggie) **SNACK #2** *(if you eat dinner late)* 2 deli roll-ups & 2 dill pickle spears
DINNER Grilled Chicken Broc w/cheese (90 cal individual svg) ½ cup brown rice **DESSERT** ¼ cup frozen dark candy pieces mixed with ½ cup Publix fro-yo, Drizzle w/0-cal chocolate sauce & top w/ lowfat whipped topping	**DINNER** 1 or 2 bags 100-cal Microwave popcorn 1 glass wine or 1 vodka/soda **Or** 1 cup whole grain cereal w/skim milk **DESSERT** 2 10-calorie gelatin dessert w/ lowfat whipped topping **Or** ½ c blueberries w/ cereal sprinkled on top, little skim milk	**DINNER** Grilled Salmon Green Beans sauteed w/ cooking spray & 1/2 tsp olive oil, few slivered almonds, sprinkle parm) 1 gl wine or 1 vodka/soda **DESSERT** Frozen bar (100 cals)

Menu: Week 2

Day Eight	Day Nine	Day Ten	Day Eleven
BREAKFAST 3 egg whites, fresh spinach, mushrooms & tomato, 1 tbsp shredded cheese 1 slice thin wheat bread w/spray butter Coffee/Tea/creamer	**BREAKFAST** Lowfat Breakfast Sandwich 1/2 c berries Coffee/Tea w/creamer	**BREAKFAST** 1 cup any whole-grain cereal w/skim or light soy milk 1/2 cup berries or 1/2 cup dark grapes Coffee / Tea w/creamer	**BREAKFAST** 100 cal English Muffin w/spray butter & sugar-free preserves 2 veggie or turkey sausages Coffee / Tea w/creamer
SNACK Small apple pre-sliced Light cheese (1 wedge or 5 cubes)	**SNACK** Nutritional Bar	**SNACK** ½ pita pocket w/few slivers sundried tomato, arugula, 2 slices deli chicken, spray 1-cal. Drsg	**SNACK** Nutritional Bar
LUNCH Small can white tuna over Huge salad with free veggies & 1-calorie drsg 16 wheat crackers	**LUNCH** 1 can low-fat soup (130 cals/serving) Huge salad 1-cal drsg 6 wheat crackers w/ 1 wedge light cheese	**LUNCH** Leftover salmon over huge salad w/1-cal drsg Small handful walnuts or almonds	**LUNCH** Diet frozen entree Huge salad w/free vegs 1-cal drsg
SNACK 100-cal snack bag **SNACK #2** *(if you eat dinner late)* 2 deli roll-ups 1 small orange	**SNACK** Antipasto with grilled peppers, marinated artichoke hearts, lunch meat, sprinkle fresh grated parm & romano **SNACK #2** *(if you eat dinner late)* 1-100 calorie yogurt sprinkled w/crunch cereal	**SNACK** 1/2 roll-up made with low-carb tortilla spread w/light cheese wedge, 2 slices deli chicken or turkey & free veggies **SNACK #2** *(if you eat dinner late)* 1 cup mixed berries w/ lowfat whipped topping	**SNACK** 2 rice cakes w/light cream cheese & strawberry slices **SNACK #2** *(if you eat dinner late)* 1-100 cal yogurt Small nectarine or plum
DINNER 1 or 2 bags 100-cal Microwave popcorn 1 cup berries (frozen or fresh) **DESSERT** 2 scoops fro-yo sundae with chocolate sauce and spray whipped cream	**DINNER** Grilled salmon w/ spinach, tomato & capers 1 cup green beans w/ spray butter & sprinkle parm 1 gl wine or 1 vodka/soda **DESSERT** ¼ cup froz. Choc. pieces & ½ cup fro-yo	**DINNER** 1 or 2 bags 100-cal Microwave popcorn **DESSERT** small cone w/appx 2 scoops fro-yo **Or** 1 60-cal gelatin dessert Pudding w/ lowfat whipped topping	**DINNER** Grilled Shrimp Roasted asparagus Salad w/arugula, few walnuts and ½ pear 1 gl wine or vod/soda **DESSERT** 1 cup frozen fresh berries or1 cup fresh fruit dipped in 0-cal chocolate sauce

Menu: Week 2

Day Twelve	Day Thirteen	Day Fourteen
BREAKFAST ½ Pita toasted w/spray butter 2 veggie or turkey sausages Coffee/Tea w/creamer	**BREAKFAST** Lowfat Breakfast Burrito Coffee / Tea w/creamer	**BREAKFAST** 3 egg whites w/ fresh spinach, tomato & 1 tbsp shredded cheese 100 cal. eng. muffin w/ SPRAY BUTTER Coffee /Tea w/creamer
SNACK Snack bag of baby carrots 5 cubes light cheese ½ Nutritional Bar	**SNACK** 1 100-calorie yogurt w/sprinkle crunchy cereal	**SNACK** 1 100-calorie yogurt w/ ½ small apple
LUNCH Huge salad w/ leftover grilled shrimp & 1-cal drsg 10 wheat crackers	**LUNCH** Leftover grilled chicken Huge salad w/1-cal drsg 1/2 sweet potato w/1 tsp light sour cream	**LUNCH** Diet frozen entree Huge salad w/1-cal drsg
SNACK Antipasto with grilled peppers, marinated artichoke hearts, lunch meat, sprinkle fresh grated parm & romano ½ small apple **SNACK #2** *(if you eat dinner late)* 1 100-calorie yogurt	**SNACK** ½ Nutritional Bar **SNACK #2** *(if you eat dinner late)* 1 cup mixed berries w/ lowfat whipped topping Light cheese (5 cubes or 1 wedge)	**SNACK** 1 cup honey nut circles (in baggie) **SNACK #2** *(if you eat dinner late)* 2 deli roll-ups 2 dill pickle spears
DINNER Grilled Chicken Broc w/cheese (90 cal individual svg) ½ cup brown rice **DESSERT** ¼ cup frozen dark M&M's mixed with ½ cup Publix fro-yo, Drizzle w/0-calorie chocolate sauce & top w/ lowfat whipped topping	**DINNER** 1 or 2 bags 100-cal Microwave popcorn 1 gl. wine or 1 vodka/soda **DESSERT** 2 10-calorie gelatin dessert w/ lowfat whipped topping **Or** ½ c blueberries w/ cereal sprinkled on top, little skim milk	**DINNER** Grilled Salmon Green Beans sauteed w/ cooking spray & 1/2 tsp olive oil, few slivered almonds, sprinkle parm) 1 gl wine or 1 vodka/soda **DESSERT** Frozen bar (100 cals)

Menu: Week 3

Day Fifteen	Day Sixteen	Day Seventeen	Day Eighteen
BREAKFAST 1 cup any whole-grain cereal w/skim or light soy milk 1/2 cup berries or 1/2 cup dark grapes Coffee / Tea w/creamer	**BREAKFAST** Lowfat Breakfast Sandwich 1/2 c berries Coffee/Tea w/creamer	**BREAKFAST** 1 cup oatmeal w/ 1/4 c skim milk & 1 cup blueberries Coffee/Tea w/creamer	**BREAKFAST** 3 egg whites w/ fresh spinach, mushrooms & tomato, 1 tbsp shredded cheese 1 slice thin wheat bread w/spray butter Coffee/Tea w/creamer
SNACK Nutritional Bar	**SNACK** Small apple pre-sliced	**SNACK** 1 cup cut melon Laughing Cow Light cheese (1 wedge / 5 cubes)	**SNACK** Fiber One, Luna or Cliff Kids Bar
LUNCH 1 lo-carb wrap spread w/1 wedge Light cheese, 1 can white tuna, free veggies & 1-calorie drsg	**LUNCH** 1 can low-fat soup (100 cals/serving) Huge salad 1-cal drsg 6 wheat crackers w/ 1 wedge Light cheese	**LUNCH** Diet frozen entree Huge salad w/1-cal drsg	**LUNCH** Diet frozen entree Huge salad w/free vegs & 1-cal drsg
SNACK 1 100-cal yogurt **SNACK #2** *(if you eat dinner late)* 2 deli roll-ups & 1 small orange	**SNACK** Antipasto with grilled peppers, marinated artichoke hearts, lunch meat, sprinkle fresh grated parm & romano **SNACK #2** *(if you eat dinner late)* 1 100-calorie yogurt sprinkled w/crunchy cereal	**SNACK** 1/2 roll-up made with low-carb tortilla, spread w/light cheese wedge, 2 slices deli chicken or turkey & free veggies **SNACK #2** *(if you eat dinner late)* 2 rice cakes w/light cream cheese & strawberry slices	**SNACK** 1 60-Calorie Soup 10 wheat crackers **SNACK #2** *(if you eat dinner late)* 1 100-cal yogurt Small nectarine or plum
DINNER 1 or 2 bags 100-cal Microwave popcorn 1 cup berries (frozen or fresh) **DESSERT** 2 scoops fro-yo sundae with 0-calorie chocolate sauce and spray whipped cream	**DINNER** Grilled Turkey Burger w/ 2 slices toasted Thin Wheat Bread spread w/1 wedge Light cheese 1/2 sweet potato wedges roasted w/ cooking spray, garlic powder & black pepper **DESSERT** 2-10 cal gelatin dessert & lowfat whipped topping	**DINNER** 1 or 2 bags 100-cal Microwave popcorn gl. Wine or 1 vodka/soda **DESSERT** small cone w/ appx 2 scoops fro-yo **Or** 1 60-cal pudding w/ lowfat whipped topping	**DINNER** Grilled Shrimp Roasted asparagus Salad w/arugula, few walnuts and ½ pear **DESSERT** 1 cup frozen fresh berries or 1 cup fresh fruit dipped in 0-calorie chocolate sauce

Menu: Week 3

Day Nineteen	Day Twenty	Day Twenty-One
BREAKFAST ½ Pita toasted w/spray butter 2 veggie or turkey sausages Coffee/Tea w/creamer	**BREAKFAST** Lowfat Breakfast Burrito Coffee / Tea w/creamer	**BREAKFAST** 1 cup oatmeal w/ 1/4 c skim milk & 1 cup blueberries Coffee /Tea w/creamer
SNACK Snack bag of baby carrots 5 cubes Light cheese ½ Nutritional Bar	**SNACK** 1 cup mixed berries w/ lowfat whipped topping	**SNACK** 1 100-calorie yogurt w/ ½ small apple
LUNCH Huge salad w/leftover grilled shrimp & 1-cal drsg 10 wheat crackers	**LUNCH** Leftover grilled chicken Huge salad w/1-cal drsg1/2 sweet potato w/1 tsp light sour cream	**LUNCH** Diet frozen entree Huge salad w/1-cal drsg
SNACK Antipasto with grilled peppers, marinated artichoke hearts, lunch meat, sprinkle fresh grated parm & romano ½ small apple **SNACK #2** *(if you eat dinner late)* 1 100-calorie yogurt	**SNACK** ½ Nutritional Bar **SNACK #2** *(if you eat dinner late)* 1 cup mixed berries w/ lowfat whipped topping Light cheese (5 cubes or 1 wedge)	**SNACK** 1 cup whole-grain cereal & small box raisins (in baggie) **SNACK#2** *(if you eat dinner late)* 2 deli roll-ups 2 dill pickle spears
DINNER Grilled Chicken Green Beans sauteed w/ cooking spray & 1/2 tsp olive oil, few slivered almonds, sprinkle parm Dinner salad w/free veggies **DESSERT** ¼ cup frozen dark choc candies mixed with ½ cup fro-yo. Drizzle w/0-calorie chocolate sauce & top w/ lowfat whipped topping	**DINNER** 1 or 2 bags 100-cal Microwave popcorn 1 gl. wine or 1 vodka/soda **DESSERT** ½ c blueberries w/cereal sprinkled on top, little skim milk	**DINNER** Grilled Salmon 1/2 sweet potato wedges roasted w/ cooking spray, garlic powder & ground pepper 1 gl wine or 1 vodka/soda **DESSERT** Frozen bar (100 cals)

Menu: Week 4

Day Twenty-Two	Day Twenty-Three	Day Twenty-Four	Day Twenty-Five
BREAKFAST 1 cup any whole-grain cereal w/skim or light soy milk 1/2 cup berries or 1/2 cup dark grapes Coffee / Tea w/creamer	**BREAKFAST** Lowfat Breakfast Sandwich 1/2 c berries Coffee/Tea w/creamer	**BREAKFAST** 1 cup oatmeal w/ 1/4 c skim milk & 1 cup blueberries Coffee/Tea w/creamer	**BREAKFAST** 3 egg whites w/ fresh spinach, mushrooms & tomato, 1 tbsp shredded cheese 1 slice thin wheat bread w/spray butter Coffee/Tea w/creamer
SNACK Nutritional Bar	**SNACK** Small apple pre-sliced	**SNACK** 1 cup cut melon Light cheese (1 wedge / 5 cubes)	**SNACK** Nutritional Bar
LUNCH 1 lo-carb wrap spread w/1 wedge Light cheese, 1 can white tuna, free veggies & 1-calorie drsg	**LUNCH** 1 can low-fat soup (100 cals/serving) Huge salad 1-cal drsg 6 WW crackers w/ 1 wedge light cheese	**LUNCH** Diet frozen entree Huge salad w/1-cal drsg	**LUNCH** Diet frozen entree Huge salad w/free vegs & 1-cal drsg
SNACK 1 100-cal yogurt **SNACK #2** *(if you eat dinner late)* 2 deli roll-ups & 1 small orange	**SNACK** Antipasto with grilled peppers, marinated artichoke hearts, lunch meat, sprinkle fresh grated parm & romano **SNACK #2** *(if you eat dinner late)* 1 100-calorie yogurt sprinkled w/ crunchy cereal	**SNACK** 1/2 roll-up made with low-carb tortilla, spread w/light cheese wedge, 2 slices deli chicken or turkey & free veggies **SNACK #2** *(if you eat dinner late)* 2 rice cakes w/light cream cheese & strawberry slices	**SNACK** 1 60-Calorie Soup 10 wheat crackers **SNACK #2** *(if you eat dinner late)* 1 100-cal yogurt Small nectarine or plum
DINNER 1 or 2 bags 100-cal Microwave popcorn 1 cup berries (frozen or fresh) **DESSERT** 2 scoops fro-yo sundae with 0-calorie chocolate sauce and spray whipped cream	**DINNER** Grilled Turkey Burger w/ 2 slices toasted thin wheat bread spread w/1 wedge light cheese 1/2 sweet potato wedges roasted w/Cooking spray, garlic powder & black pepper **DESSERT** **2-10 cal gelatin desserts & lowfat whipped topping**	**DINNER** 1 or 2 bags 100-cal Microwave popcorn gl. Wine or 1 vodka/soda **DESSERT** small cone w/ appx 2 scoops fro-yo **Or** 1 60-cal pudding w/ lowfat whipped topping	**DINNER** Grilled Shrimp Roasted asparagus Salad w/arugula, few walnuts and 1/2 pear **DESSERT** 1 cup frozen fresh berries or 1 cup fresh fruit dipped in 0-calorie chocolate sauce

52

Menu: Week 4

Day Twenty-Six	Day Twenty-Seven	Day Twenty-Eight
BREAKFAST ½ Pita toasted w/spray butter 2 veggie or turkey sausages Coffee/Tea w/creamer	**BREAKFAST** Lowfat Breakfast Burrito Coffee / Tea w/creamer	**BREAKFAST** 1 cup oatmeal w/ 1/4 c skim milk & 1 cup blueberries Coffee /Tea w/creamer
SNACK Snack bag of baby carrots 5 cubes Light cheese ½ Nutritional Bar	**SNACK** 1 cup mixed berries w/ lowfat whipped topping	**SNACK** 1 100-calorie yogurt w/ ½ small apple
LUNCH Huge salad w/leftover grilled shrimp & 1-cal drsg 10 wheat crackers	**LUNCH** Leftover grilled chicken Huge salad w/1-cal drsg1/2 sweet potato w/1 tsp light sour cream	**LUNCH** Diet frozen entree Huge salad w/1-cal drsg
SNACK Antipasto with grilled peppers, marinated artichoke hearts, lunch meat, sprinkle fresh grated parm & romano ½ small apple **SNACK #2** *(if you eat dinner late)* 1 100-calorie yogurt	**SNACK** ½ Nutritional Bar **SNACK #2** *(if you eat dinner late)* 1 cup mixed berries w/ lowfat whipped topping Light cheese (5 cubes or 1 wedge)	**SNACK** 1 cup whole-grain cereal & small box raisins (in baggie) **SNACK#2** *(if you eat dinner late)* 2 deli roll-ups 2 dill pickle spears
DINNER Grilled Chicken Green Beans sauteed w/ cooking spray & 1/2 tsp olive oil, few slivered almonds, sprinkle parm Dinner salad w/free veggies **DESSERT** ¼ cup frozen dark choc pieces mixed with ½ cup Publix fro-yo. Drizzle w/0-calorie chocolate sauce & top w/ lowfat whipped topping	**DINNER** 1 or 2 bags 100-cal Microwave popcorn 1 gl. wine or 1 vodka/soda **DESSERT** ½ c blueberries w/cereal sprinkled on top, little skim milk	**DINNER** Grilled Salmon 1/2 sweet potato wedges roasted w/ cooking spray, garlic powder & ground pepper 1 gl wine or 1 vodka/soda **DESSERT** Frozen bar (100 cals)

SAMPLE MENU with notes

Here's a typical day's menu with my notes/tips.

Breakfast

¾ c oatmeal with skim or light soy milk if desired

½ c berries or ½ c dark grapes

Coffee / tea / me ☺

NOTE: when I first started losing, I would add a little flavored creamer because I liked it. I've evolved now to doing coffee with 2 whatever artificial sweeteners I have on hand. If you're a big fan of the newer, naturally-derived sweeteners, go for it! Unlike the pink stuff, it isn't alleged to cause cancer in laboratory rats.

I also squirt about 2 tbsp of whatever kind of whipped cream I have in the fridge – no sugar added, heavy, whatever – they're all around 20 calories per 2 tbsp. Knock yourself out.

Snack

(appx. 1-2 hours later)

½ Nutritional Bar

Or

Kid-sized nutritional bar

NOTE: Kid versions of nutritional bars have about 100 fewer calories than the adult ones.

Lunch

1 low-carb wrap with 1 slice light cheese, 1 small can white tuna in water & all the veggies you can pack into the wrap. I like shredded carrots, onions (unless I have a date later), leafy lettuces, broccoli slaw (plain), cukes, tomatoes – pile 'em on.

Spray of 1-calorie dressing

¼ sliced avocado

Snack (appx. 2 hours later)

100-calorie yogurt

NOTE: I love doing the vanilla one, and tossing in several berries.

Sometimes I even freeze it a little – it changes the texture, and I'm a texture-holic.

Snack (appx. 2 hours later)

1 oz sliced grilled chicken (I buy mine already grilled, or do leftover grilled chicken. I like it cold. Like my men.)

1 small orange

¼ c almonds or walnuts

Dinner

Salmon prepared with olive oil cooking spray, capers, fresh spinach leaves and sun-dried tomatoes

½ c long grain brown rice seasoned with fresh Parmesan

1 c berries

NOTE: I get a 6 oz. piece of fresh salmon, and I make the whole thing at once but only eat 3 oz. and save the rest for next day.

Spray pan with cooking spray; put salmon skin-side up in hot pan. Flip it when it's opaque half-way thru; turn it over; throw in capers (they pop and get crunchy when you cook them – imagine that!), spinach leaves and sun-dried tomatoes. Cook till salmon is opaque all the way thru. You'll think you're dining in a fancy restaurant. You can thank me later.

Dessert

2 scoops frozen yogurt sundae with 0-calorie chocolate sauce and whipped light cream

CHAPTER SEVEN
A La Carte Menu

While some of you might like the 28-day, fixed menu plan, some of you might like to pick and choose your meals. So have at it, my friend. Have at it.

You will be fluctuating your caloric intake from about 1,100 to 1,600 a day – 75- to 150-calorie mini-meals, with higher-calorie meals when you want them. I also think one reason I had success NOT doing a traditional "1,400 calorie a day diet" was because I made my body guess from day to day what it was getting…

The way I designed it is that you shouldn't worry about eating everything for the day if you're not hungry! There will be days you're naturally more hungry, or you have parties, or you still turn to food for comfort (like me, you may have spent most of your life using food for uses other than what it was intended), and those habits die hard. I still have to stop and register whether I'm hungry or just going thru something and that's why I'm turning to food. Conversely, there will be days you're either less physically hungry, or busier. The goal is to eat every 2 or so hours…therefore, you're never hungry.

I want you to actually eat before you're starving, which is a surefire way to make you eat something you know you don't really want, but it's there, so – hey – why not? Note: these quick go-to's are RARELY what you really want – they're usually the crust of your kid's

PB&J, or stale cookies from the office jar, or a slimy fast-food cheeseburger derived from God Knows What.

Think about your reasons for wanting this to be the last time you ever need to even THINK about losing weight – once you're at your goal, you will NEVER HAVE TO DO IT AGAIN. Truthfully, how I ate to lose my 55 pounds is how I mostly still eat today – it makes my body feel great, and if I want something allegedly "naughty," I have it. But I'm not tempted to overindulge – ever – because I feel so fabulous physically, and mentally, it changed my life - because I never want to have to worry about having to lose weight again. The maintenance of this approach is laughably easy. You will see!

Note: as I'm finishing this chapter, my kids came home from a birthday party and brought home a leftover pizza from a chain. I wasn't really hungry, but today I'm stressed a bit, finishing up this chapter, so without thinking I downed a piece of cold, congealed pizza. I don't even LIKE chain pizza! I'm a pizza snob from Jersey! Yet, I did it. And how do I feel right now? Bloated. Kind of mad at myself for eating without thinking. But it's ok – we are human and we will ALL always have times like this. I will use this as a note to self – I feel physically not good – it's not a crime to have eaten the slice – but before I was even done, I was already thinking "wow, this doesn't even taste good. Why am I eating this? And I wonder how many 10 year olds sneezed on this before I'm now chewing it?" So, yeah, think before you stuff. But what's funny is that if were the "old me" – I would instead be thinking "Well, I blew it, so now I'll go raid the fridge and pantry and get my fill of whatever I think I can't have tomorrow – when I'll try to be back 'on' my 'diet'"– thereby feeling even sicker, fuller, and more and more disgusted with myself.

Instead, I will drink green tea – that will alleviate my belly bloat, and get me immediately over the guilts and back in a good head-space. If I eat anything else tonight (which I probably won't – it's late), it will be a piece of fruit or a 10-calorie frozen bar. So there.

Breakfast Options

I like to keep it around 200-250 calories. Use your judgment based on whether you're in a hurry, have to eat on the fly, are having breakfast out, have to run through a drive-thru, etc. Pick these meals and mini-meals based on what's a practical fit with your lifestyle on any particular day. But be sure to eat in the morning!

1. Any lowfat breakfast sandwich
2. English muffin egg sandwich – take the Canadian bacon off of it, or just eat half the bacon – it will reduce your calories down to around 200.
3. ½ Pita toasted with spray butter & 2 veggie or turkey sausages
4. 100-calorie English muffin with spray butter & 1 veggie or turkey sausage
5. 3 egg whites made with Cooking spray, fresh spinach, tomato & 1 tsp shredded cheese & 1 slice thin wheat toast with spray butter

6. ¾ cup oatmeal with ¼ c. skim milk & 1 cup berries

7. ½ whole grain pita pocket containing 2 veggie or turkey sausage and 2 egg whites scrambled with Cooking spray and ½ slice light cheese

8. 1 cup cereal with ¼ c. skim milk

   Note: In theory, you could have whatever kind of cereal you want, but I stick to the ones that are highest in fiber and protein and lower in sugar…pay attention to serving size! I was never so sad the day I actually went to the trouble of measuring out a cup of whatever it was I was eating – much to my dismay, I'd been thinking a cup was much much larger than it actually is! You're only tricking yourself if you eyeball measurements incorrectly.

9. 1 thin bagel or ½ regular bagel, scooped out, toasted, with a tbsp of any kind of cream cheese, tomato, onion (if you like), and 1 oz. smoked salmon or lox. If you skip the fish, you should have a turkey or veggie sausage so you're not all-carbs.

10. 2 slices of whole-grain toast and a turkey or veggie sausage

11. 1 slice whole-grain toast with 3 scrambled egg whites with cheese & veggies

12. 1 slice French toast with spray butter and lite syrup (watch your serving size!) & ½ cup berries

13. 1 poached egg with 2 slices thin wheat toast with spray butter & 1 turkey or veggie sausage

Lunch or Dinner Options

These are around 240-350 calories each.

Key to dinner is LOAD UP ON STEAMED AND GRILLED VEGGIES – NO ONE EVER GOT FAT EATING TOO MANY VEGGIES!

1. Extra-crunchy chicken coating prepared as packaged - use 4 oz. Protein (chicken) as your portion size. Add cup & 1/4 of whatever fresh veggies and a big salad or 1/4 c. brown rice, seasoned or ½ sweet potato made into fries (see recipe section).

2. Shrimp sautéed in tsp olive oil with garlic cloves & fresh tomato; when it's done, toss in a few fresh veggies like small broccoli or baby green beans for color & crunch. Top with a tsp. of goat cheese or blue cheese for added flavor, throw a few slivered almonds or walnut pieces on top. If you want, have with 1/4 cup whole wheat pasta. Have with a giant baby green salad or Caesar lite (from bagged salad - try to avoid using the croutons, it's not worth the extra calories - get your crunch from the nuts instead).

3. Chicken salad made with grilled cold chicken or canned white meat chicken (3 oz.), a few slices of grapes & apples (Granny Smiths are good because they're tart in this), a tsp. walnuts, and ½ cup non-fat plain yogurt (50 calories' worth). Put in a giant hollowed-out tomato & have with a

side salad and a few low-fat wheat crackers or crisp bread spread with light cheese wedge.

4. Grilled Sea Bass (4 oz.) (or salmon, or any fish you like) over morel mushrooms & mashed sweet potato (with spray butter & 1 teaspoon light sour cream) with a side salad & 1 1/4 cups fresh veggies like green beans or broccoli.

5. Grilled salmon (6 oz., have half today and half for lunch or dinner tomorrow): Cooking spray spray; 6 oz. salmon, skin on. Heat skillet, cook salmon til halfway opaque; flip; add capers, spinach, tomatoes…cook til firm and opaque throughout. Have with a giant portion of whatever veggies you like, fresh, raw, steamed or grilled. If you like, add a sprinkle of a really good Parmesan cheese to the veggies – they're so low in calories, you can jazz them up with a little cheese to make them seem more delicious!

Tip: Get mango salsa if you can - it's only about 20 calories for 2 tbsp. and you can add it to any fish or chicken dish you make - it's a lot of flavor for barely any calories!

6. Spaghetti squash (if you haven't tried it, try it, it's fabulous) with garlic, olive oil & pine nuts, with a giant green salad or light Caesar salad. Have a slice of whole-grain bread with 1 teaspoon almond butter if you need an additional bread with this.

7. Chicken baked with low-sodium mushroom soup (again, make 6 oz. and eat the rest the following day), ½ c brown rice, giant salad and veggies

8. Grilled or baked chicken or meat (6 oz., eat half at this meal and the other half at lunch or dinner tomorrow – are you catching a pattern here? ☺) Green beans sautéed with ½ tsp olive oil or olive oil spritz, a few slivered almonds, a sprinkle of parm.

9. Ginormous salad

10. Grilled Turkey Burger: 2 slices toasted wheat thin bread or any low-carb, low-calorie bun (keep the calories per serving under 100), 1 thin slice any cheese, ½ sweet potato wedges

11. Apricot chicken (6 oz. chicken – 3 oz. this meal, 3 oz. tomorrow), 1 tsp. low-calorie, no-sugar apricot preserves mixed w/ ½ tsp. dried minced onion & thinly spread over chicken and then baked til chicken done, 1 cup any veggies

12. Grilled Shrimp, roasted veggies, salad with arugula, ¼ c walnuts, ½ pear, & 1 tsp. blue cheese crumbles

13. Diet frozen entree under 320 calories

I'm a big fan of the 180-calorie turkey and sweet potato one, and the 250-calorie turkey and stuffing and green beans one - the pizzas are also yummy, as are the Mexican selections. Always add tons of veggies and/or a salad to these, depending on how your appetite is.

Vegetarian selections rock, too – watch the calories – just because it's extremely healthy doesn't necessarily mean it's low-calorie!

With my lifestyle, I tend to rely on frozen dinners and lunches a few times a week. Plus, I'm a terrible cook – just ask my kids. Or my ex-husband ☺ There's no harm in eating them, as long as you don't have to restrict your sodium. Fortunately, even if you do, you can find many selections now that are lower in sodium than they used to be.

Mini-Meal Options

To be eaten about 2 hours after breakfast and lunch (will be about 75-150 calories)

1. Nutritional bar
2. 1 cup berries with a FEW walnuts or almonds
3. Snack bag of baby carrots with 5 cubes or 1 wedge of light cheese
4. 100-calorie yogurt w/sprinkle of Crunchy cereal
5. Small apple with light cheese wedge spread on it
6. Small apple with 1 tsp peanut butter
7. ½ pita pocket with a few slivers of sundried tomato, shredded carrots, arugula leaves, 2 slices deli chicken or turkey, spritz with a few sprays of 1-calorie salad dressing. I like higher-quality deli meats because I'm also a deli snob. No, seriously, it'll taste better, and isn't that what it's all about- stuff tasting good?
8. 1 bag 100-calorie popcorn
9. 100-calorie snack packs – try not to depend on these – I'd rather you ate fruits, proteins and veggies – so limit these carby treats to only a few a week. You will start seeing how much better you feel – with more energy! When you eat more fruits and veggies, you'll want the junk food less and you'll crave the good stuff – I'm serious!
10. ¼ c frozen dark chocolate pieces with ½ cup low-fat frozen yogurt

11. 2 deli meat roll-ups (whatever kind of meat you like) – 2 oz. – made with 1-calorie salad dressing, heart of palm, sun dried tomatoes and a small nectarine

12. Antipasto with grilled peppers, marinated artichoke hearts, deli meat (2 oz.), sprinkle freshly grated parm cheese, ½ small apple

13. An orange and a few dry-roasted nuts

14. 10 cashew nuts

15. 10 almonds

16. Half a small avocado

17. 3 ounces cooked whole-grain noodles with 1 fresh tomato and 1/2 ounce hard cheese

18. 1 seven-grain Belgian waffle

19. 4 mini rice cakes with 2 tablespoons low-fat cottage cheese

20. 3 ounces low-fat cottage cheese and 3 whole-wheat crackers

21. 1/4 cup fat-free ranch dressing with mixed raw veggies

22. 6 wheat crackers with two teaspoons of peanut butter (or any nut butter)

23. 1 small baked potato with 1/2 cup salsa and 2 tablespoons of fat-free sour cream

24. 1/3 cup of unsweetened applesauce with 1 slice of whole-wheat toast, cut into 4 strips for dunking

25. 1/2 cup frozen orange juice, eaten as sorbet

26. 2 large graham cracker squares with 1 teaspoon peanut butter

27. 3 handfuls of unbuttered popcorn, seasoned with herbs

28. A 5-ounce tossed salad with lettuce, tomato, cucumber and 1/4 cup fat-free dressing

29. Half a "finger" of string cheese with 4 whole-wheat crackers

CHAPTER EIGHT

Calorie Counts on Good-For-You Foods

Fruits – Servings & Calories

Blackberries	1 cup	90 calories
Blueberries	1 cup	80 calories
Cantaloupe	1 cup cubed	55 calories
Apple	1 medium	80 calories
Apple Sauce,		
Sweetened	½ cup	100 calories
Unsweetened	½ cup	60 calories
Apricots, fresh	1 medium	20 calories
Banana	1 small	90 calories
Clementines	1 small	35 calories
Cherries,		
sweet, fresh with pits	½ cup	45 calories
Figs, fresh	1 medium	35 calories
Grapefruit	½ medium	40 calories
Grapes, Red or Green	10 grapes	35 calories
Honeydew Melon	1 cup cubed	60 calories
Kiwi	1 medium	45 calories
Mandarin Oranges,		
canned, drained	1 cup	70 calories
Mango, thinly sliced	½ cup	55 calories

Nectarine	1 medium	65 calories
Orange	1 medium	65 calories
Papaya	1 cup sliced	55 calories
Peach	1 medium	40 calories
Pear	1 medium	100 calories
Pineapple, fresh	1 cup	75 calories
Raspberries	1 cup	60 calories
Strawberries	1 cup	50 calories
Tangerine	1 medium	35 calories
Watermelon, diced	1 cup	45 calories

Fruit can be a good source of fiber. Both the fiber and the high water content of fruit can work together to keep you from feeling hungry. Not all fruits are equally good sources of fiber, though. As a general rule the best sources include the berries, citrus fruits (eaten whole not as juice), and fruit eaten with the skin such as pears and apples.

Vegetables – Servings & Calories

Acorn squash	½ cup, cooked	57 calories
Artichokes	½ cup, cooked	42 calories
Asparagus	½ cup, cooked	23 calories
Beets	½ cup, cooked	26 calories
Black beans	1 cup, cooked	227 calories
Broccoli – chopped	1 cup, cooked	22 calories
Brussel sprouts	1 cup, cooked	30 calories

Butterhead lettuce	1 cup, raw	5 calories
Butternut squash	½ cup, cooked	41 calories
Cabbage	1 cup, cooked	16 calories
Capers	1 tbsp	5 calories
Carrots	1 carrot	31 calories
(individual bag of baby carrots)		35 calories
Cauliflower, raw	3 florets	13 calories
Celery	½ cup, raw	10 calories
Chives – raw	1 tablespoon	1 calorie
Corn	1 ear	80 calories
Cucumbers	½, raw	20 calories
Eggplant	½ cup, raw	13 calories
Garbanzo beans	1 cup, cooked	286 calories
Garlic	1 clove	4 calories
Green beans	1 cup, raw	34 calories
Green peas	1 cup, cooked	67 calories
Iceberg lettuce	1 cup, raw	18 calories
Kidney beans	1 cup, cooked	215 calories
Lentils	1 cup, cooked	226 calories
Lima beans	1 cup, cooked	190 calories
Mushrooms	½ cup, raw	21 calories
Mustard greens	½ cup, raw	15 calories
Navy beans	1 cup, cooked	296 calories
Okra	½ cup, raw	26 calories
Onions	½ cup, raw	30 calories
Parsley	½ cup, raw	10 calories

Peppers, green or red	½ cup, raw	14 calories
Pickles	Check variety between 0 & 5 calories	
Pinto beans	1 cup, cooked	206 calories
Potatoes	1 7-oz, raw	220 calories
Pumpkin	½ cup, cooked	41 calories
Radish	½ cup, raw	10 calories
Rhubarb	1 cup, raw	26 calories
Romaine lettuce	1 cup, raw	9 calories
Scallions	½ cup, raw	16 calories
Spinach	1 cup, cooked	20 calories
Sweet potatoes	1 4-oz., raw	117 calories
Tomatoes, raw	1 4-oz	26 calories
Turnips	½ cup, boiled	14 calories
Yellow squash	½ cup, raw	14 calories
Zucchini	½ cup, raw	14 calories

CHAPTER NINE
Vegetarian Options

Vegetarian Choices – you can substitute any protein (3-4 oz.) to replace the obvious "veggie" items (i.e. use turkey bacon or turkey sausage; or use chicken in place of shrimp if you choose, etc.)

Breakfast Options

1. Egg white & asparagus omelet cooked w/ olive oil spray or a teaspoon of olive oil. You can add a tablespoon of any cheese you want. Have one slice of whole grain bread or a pita, not to exceed 100 calories for the bread; spread with the spray butter. You can use 3 or 4 egg whites or egg white substitute equivalent. Add 2 veggie sausages. You can substitute asparagus for spinach or broccoli, too.

2. Oatmeal with berries & 2 veggie sausages

3. French toast made with 2 slices whole grain bread (not to exceed 150 calories total for bread) - you can even use a slice of raisin bread, but only one slice - it's around 100 calories for 1 slice of raisin bread. Use only egg whites or egg white substitute. Top w/light syrup, have a tablespoon of almonds or walnuts with it, and 1 veggie sausage.

4. Breakfast burrito made with egg substitute or egg whites, veggie sausage or veggie bacon & 1 tablespoon cheese in a low-carb wrap (wrap shouldn't exceed 100 calories). Have a cup of fresh berries or a small orange too.

Lunch Options

1. Broiled or grilled shrimp with a mixed green salad with a teaspoon of blue cheese or goat cheese, and 1-calorie spray-on dressing; and a sliced pear.

2. Pita pocket (80 calories maximum) stuffed with tuna (3 oz. can). Spread pita with dijon or yellow mustard, stuff also with as many veggies as you can get in there! Or make the tuna & stuff into a hollowed-out big tomato. Have 10 low-fat wheat crackers with this unless you have the pita, then don't have the crackers.

3. Strawberries and cottage cheese (60 calorie-little cup cottage cheese, 1 cup strawberries, 1 tablespoon almonds) and a grilled cheese & tomato sandwich (1 slice Swiss or American cheese, tomato slices, and 2 slices very thin wheat bread (3=110 calories, just have 2 slices). Open-faced in toaster oven or broiler, or grilled with spray butter or olive oil spray.

4. Veggie Bacon, Lettuce & Tomato Sandwich on thin wheat bread, 1 teaspoon low-calorie mayo or mustard, as much tomato & lettuce as you can fit onto the sandwich. 1 bag 100 calorie chips, any kind. 1/2 cup berries or a small piece of fruit, like a nectarine or orange.

CHAPTER TEN

Dining Out: Guide to Healthy Eating in a Cesspool of Fat

I always eat something before I head out the door – usually a cup of steamed green beans (hot or cold) at about 30 calories; or a half a cut-up apple. You'd be surprised how filling they are! Remember too that it takes at least 20 minutes for your belly to signal your brain that it's full. By the time you get to the restaurant, you will be able to take it easy with your portions, because you'll already be somewhat satisfied hunger-wise!

ITALIAN

If you go to an Italian restaurant, try and structure the meal they do in Italy – in courses, with a modest serving of al dente pasta topped with a healthy tomato sauce, followed by a main course of fish, poultry or meat and fresh vegetables (including either leafy green ones like escarole or spinach, or crucifers like broccoli) – plus a salad dressing in olive oil and balsamic vinegar. Also, you can have an antipasto as your meal!

In Italy, you don't sit down in front of a huge dish of pasta with a bottomless breadbasket and call it dinner. That's why Italians can typically eat pasta twice a day and not suffer the obesity rates we see in the United States.

Request Half-Orders

You can request a half-order of pasta as your appetizer in many restaurants. If you try this, you'll see that it satisfies. It's important to eat enough good fats (the entrée and the olive oil) to counter the starches in the pasta.

ASIAN

We all tend to assume that Asian restaurants are serving healthy food. The various Asian national diets tend to be heavy on fish, seafood & veggies, light on heavy meats and sweets. But that's not always the case in Asian restaurants in America. Here are the things to watch out for:

Oversized Portions

One major difference is portion size – we are accustomed to a lot more food on our plates. And because everybody hates waste, we tend to finish what's there.

Bad Carbs

Another significant difference is in the rice. Asians have always used the whole grain, including the fiber, which requires the digestive system to work harder to get at the starch. In this country, and increasingly in many Asian cities, a more processed variety of white rice is used. That change substantially increases the glycemic load of a meal. I suggest staying away from rice altogether. Instead, order a double serving of veggies, or limit portions of rice by eating servings no bigger than a tennis ball at most. Another trick I employ is always ordering a small serving of Miso soup – very filling and healthy.

Hidden sugars

Something else you may not realize is that MSG, the flavoring agent, is made from beets. The beet is a healthy vegetable, but it has a very high glycemic index. Beets are loaded with sugar, but disguised fairly well in your average Chinese take-out dinner. Many people are also sensitive to MSG. Request the MSG to be left out of your dish- if it's a good restaurant, you won't notice the omission.

Sushi!!!! Saved me for most of my weight-loss phase and now my maintenance! Again, avoid rice whenever possible! The seaweed salad is a great choice, as are any of the raw fish selections. Also wonderful are the salmon rolls (with seaweed or thin rice paper outside, julienned cucumbers, carrots & spicy wasabi sauce on the inside) or shrimp or summer rolls. The sushi roll menu is usually extensive.

Try to stay away from anything "tempura" – or share it with a dining companion if you really really want it. Opt for Miso soup, a salad with a small amount of ginger dressing, and several selections of sushi (without the rice, or with much of the rice knocked off of it – I do this all the time). Sushi is very filling, flavorful, and colorful, and I never feel too full or at all guilty when I walk out of a sushi restaurant! Even most grocery stores now have sushi in their prepared food section.

One other startling observation I made the last time I was eating hibachi-style at our local sushi / Asian restaurant: We had ordered salmon & shrimp (sounds healthy, right)? Then the chef did his little magic show, and when he commenced cooking, he loaded about a half-pound of butter on top of the salmon, shrimp and veggies! I can't even imagine how much fat and how many calories were added to an otherwise healthy choice.

GREEK OR MIDDLE EASTERN

Going to Greek or Middle Eastern restaurants is a great choice because these cuisines employ lots of olive oil – always a plus. You can have hummus (paste made from chickpeas) on pita bread, which is a big improvement over white bread and butter, and it's more flavorful, too. You'll find good, whole grains such as tabbouleh and couscous, which take the place of potatoes or rice. These cuisines usually rely on spices and condiments rather than sweeteners to flavor the dishes. I happen to really love grape leaves – ask and see what they're stuffed with – sometimes it's just veggies, other times meats and rice – opt for the veggie-stuffed ones whenever possible. Highly flavorful and fun to eat! Also, load up on salads drizzled with olive oil.

AMERICAN

A cheeseburger, French fries, and a sugary soda may be the pinnacle of American cuisine (yikes, how did that happen?) Here's how to eat it right:

Have a burger made from a good cut of meat, like sirloin, or opt for a turkey or veggie burger.

Instead of a bun, have it on whole-wheat pita or sourdough bread, or better yet, skip the bun (or have only half a bun).

Watch for hidden sauces; ask for yours plain and then add a little mustard & ketchup if you like it.

Load your burger up with lettuce, tomato, pickles & onion.

Fries are not a good idea – steal a few from your dining partner if you must, but savor them and remind yourself of the reasons you're staying in control! Potato chips are actually a wiser choice, provided you stick to a very small amount (10 potato chips generally equal 100 calories). French-fried sweet potatoes are a better choice than either – if cooked in a monounsaturated oil. Best choice: cole slaw (as long as its not drenched in mayo) and/or a salad.

DESSERT

No news flash on this one – I do the three-bite rule, if I order it at all. I usually have a glass of wine instead. If I have a sweet craving later, I have a 10-calorie gelatin dessert with whipped cream on top, or a no-sugar added fudge pop (40 calories!) or a 60-calorie pudding. I am never hungry after dinner and before dessert comes, so if I use my head, do I really need that dessert? Chances are good that the answer is no – but if it is YES, and you're being social, go ahead and have a couple of bites – enjoy it, but don't regret. A really good dessert at a nice restaurant is not usually an every-day occurrence for most people, and the majority of your eating will be on your terms where you are choosing the right foods. So go ahead and indulge once in a while – it's the sum of the parts, done consistently, that both form healthy habits and keep you on course to lose weight every week! And remember, desserts are best shared.

GENERAL NOTES

You can log onto www.calorie-count.com and plug in all sorts of brand-name foods and also restaurant chains – I plugged in info for one popular steak house chain at the request of a client one time, and was amazed (and saddened!) to see how way off-base I'd been all those times I'd ordered grilled chicken or grilled shrimp, only to see that the calories were about 3 times what I had thought they would be! Restaurants customarily drench their grilled choices in butter and oils during preparation! If you do order grilled seafood or chicken at any restaurant, please tell the waiter you want your food "seasoned only- no butter" – they will be happy to comply and you'll be happy with your scale!

Along those lines, ask the server to prepare veggies WITHOUT butter – only seasoning!

Try just having an appetizer, and ask the server to only bring you half your entrée and ask them to package up the rest for you to take home – or better yet, share!

Fill up on salad and balsamic vinegar with a tiny bit of olive oil.

You can have bread, but just have a little.

Pizza – try having just one slice and a giant salad. You'll be full.

Remember, if you eat out constantly, because of your job or other factors, don't act as if every restaurant meal is your last. You can almost never go wrong with ordering chicken or fish prepared without butter or sauce, some veggies (also with no butter or sauce), and a big salad (remember the O&V on the side). You can always take home the extra chicken or fish for the next day.

Regarding beverages: Water water water – iced tea – diet soda if you must – never a sugary beverage! *So* not worth the calories – you're dining out, and you'd rather use those calories on food!

Regarding alcohol: Remember, each 4 oz. glass of wine is between 80 and 110 calories. Champagne actually has about 10-20 fewer calories per glass! Beer typically has between 70 and 120 calories per 8 oz.; shots of alcohol (vodka, rum, etc.) have about 100 calories each…so, the best choices for lower-calorie drinks are champagne, beer, wine, and mixed drinks (like vodka and tonic or soda; rum and diet coke; gin and tonic). Beware margaritas!!! A margarita on the rocks can have 600 calories or more PER DRINK!!! Likewise for most frozen drinks and white Russian-type drinks. Please save these for special occasions!!! (See next chapter for more info).

CHAPTER ELEVEN
Alcohol- To Drink or Not To Drink?

No matter what your poison, remember one rule of thumb: the higher the alcohol content, the higher the calories.

For example, 80-proof vodka (40% alcohol, the most common type) has 64 calories per ounce. 100-proof vodka, on the other hand, (50% alcohol) has 82 calories per ounce.

Like food portions, the calorie count of wine and alcoholic beverages is based upon a smaller serving size than what you often consume. Beer servings, however, are more standardized in bottles and beer glasses (unless you are into doing keg stands).

The average glass of wine contains 125-150 calories, but this can vary depending on the size of the glass and how full it is. What makes it even more difficult to count calories and track your alcohol consumption is that when you're out at a party or a restaurant, your glass is often refilled before it's even empty. While this bottomless glass of alcohol seems like a good idea at the time, it will not only increase your chance of a hangover, it will also lower your inhibitions in terms of how much food you consume along with your drink. This lowering of inhibitions may also lead to an unfortunate "coyote" moment the morning after.

A 12-ounce serving of beer can range anywhere from 64-198 calories. Light beers (now often popularly referred to as "low-carb" beers) contain the same amount of alcohol as regular beers, but are often lower in calories and carbohydrates than their "regular" counterparts. For example, a regular 12-oz. Budweiser is 145 calories while its counterpart, Bud Light, clocks in at a mere 110. And the superlight Bud Select is a sweet 99. (Shout out to my bro in law Jeff - you can thank me later).

You also need to be super-leery of the new popular "dessert cocktails." You know the ones I'm talking about. They beckon to you from the menu with ingredients like chocolate, buttered rum, and cream. Some of them have more calories than a real dessert. If you want to indulge in one, see if you can convince the bartender to substitute other ingredients for the really fattening ones (see tips below).

So how do you keep those calories in alcoholic drinks from adding up so quickly? Here are five tips that I've culled from the experts.

1. **Alternate between alcoholic and nonalcoholic drinks**. After that first *aaaah* glass of wine, beer or cocktail, switch to a "mocktail"- a calorie-free, nonalcoholic beverage (think sparkling water with a twist of lemon or lime) that looks real but won't weigh you down. This will not only keep you from drinking too much, it will also help you stay hydrated. Or, start your evening with the "mocktail" to help fill you up and stave off thirst.

2. **Choose wine, light beer, or simple cocktails made with low-calorie mixers**. Be friends with your bartender. Ask him or her to mix your drink using water, club soda, artificial sweeteners, or sugar-free syrup. For example, choosing diet soda over regular can save you at least 50 calories if you have it as your mixer in even just one drink. Fruit and vegetable juices are good choices because they are lower in calories than some other mixers and also contain antioxidants. But they are often high in sugar and can have a lot of "hidden" calories. Request lower-calorie juices instead.

Below are some mixers that won't pack on the pounds:
- Diet soda or diet tonic: 0 calories
- Orange juice (6 oz): 84 calories
- Cranberry juice cocktail (8 oz): 136 calories
- Light orange juice (8 oz): 50 calories
- Light cranberry juice (8 oz): 40 calories
- Light lemonade (8 oz): 5 calories
- Coffee, tea: 0 calories
- Sugar-free margarita or sweet 'n' sour mix: 0 calories
- Lemon or lime juice (1/2 oz): 10 calories
- Sugar-free syrups: 0

3. **Skip the mixer.** There are some new flavored liquors that you can order on the rocks, no mixer needed. Infused

vodkas, for example, are not sweetened but infused with flavors, from jalapeno to peach. This adds flavor without extra calories.

4. **Dilute your drink**. Club soda or sparkling water can be used to dilute your drink without taking away flavor. Think wine spritzers, which can cut the calories in a glass of wine by half. And if you usually indulge in a mixed drink like vodka and cranberry or vodka and O.J., try it with club soda, a splash of cranberry or orange juice, and a squeeze of lime. Garnishing with a wedge of citrus or pineapple adds flavor with few calories.

5. **Make a game plan.** Like making food choices in advance, having a plan before you go out to that bar or party is imperative. Decide the number of cocktails you are going to allow yourself, and make your food choices throughout the day accordingly. Do eat one of your allowed snacks before you go out. This will keep you from getting tipsy with the first drink and keep you less tempted from diving headfirst into the food. As with any other indulgence, be aware of your own personal limits. Don't drink too much, and, of course, don't drink and drive.

Some lower-calorie choices (less than 150 calories/serving):
- Alcohol-free wine (5 oz): 20-30

- Bloody Mary (5 oz): 118
- Champagne (5oz): 106-120
- Fuzzy Navel (4 oz.) has 120 calories
- Green apple martini (1 oz each vodka, sour apple, apple juice): 148
- Light beer (12 oz): 95-136
- Manhattan (2.5 oz.) : 130
- Hard Lemonade (11 oz): 98
- Mimosa (4 oz): 75
- Port wine (3 oz):128
- Red wine (5 oz):120
- Rum and Diet Coke (8 oz): 100
- Skinnygirl margarita (4 oz): 100
- Sloe Gin Fizz (8 oz.): 120
- Spiced cider with rum (8 oz):150
- Tom Collins (7.5 oz.) : 120
- Ultra-light beer (12 oz): 64-95
- White wine (5 oz): 120
- Wine spritzer (5 oz): 100

Some higher-calories choices (ask your bartender to substitute ingredients, or refrain entirely):
- Beer (12 oz): 150-198
- Chocolate martini: (2 oz each vodka, chocolate liqueur, cream, 1/2 oz creme de cacao, chocolate syrup): 438

- Coffee liqueur (3 ounces): 348
- Cosmopolitan (4 oz): 200 calories
- Eggnog with rum (8 ounces): 370
- Gin and tonic (7 oz): 200
- Chocolate liqueur (3 oz): 310
- Hot buttered rum (8 oz): 292
- Hot chocolate with peppermint schnapps (8 oz): 380
- Long Island iced tea (8 oz): 780
- Mai Tai (6 oz) (1.5 oz rum, 1/2 oz cream de along, 1/2 oz triple sec, sour mix, pineapple juice): 350
- Margarita (8 oz): 280
- Martini (2.5 oz): 160
- Mojito (8 oz): 214 calories
- Mulled wine (5 oz): 200
- Pina Colada (6 oz): 378 calories
- Rum and Coke (8 oz): 185
- Screwdriver (8 oz): 190
- Vodka and tonic (8 oz): 200
- White Russian (2 oz vodka, 1.5 oz coffee liqueur, 1.5 oz cream): 425

Low Calorie Alcoholic Drinks #1—Vodka Tonic or Gin & Tonic

Both vodka and gin have 64 calories per ounce, but it's the mixers people have with them that can pack on calories. Even if you did straight shots of them, one shot glass is 2 ounces, so that's 128 calories every time you throw your head back.

The best way to turn vodka or gin into low calorie alcoholic drinks is to just add diet tonic water and a wedge of lemon or lime. 1.5 oz. vodka or gin (96) + 4 oz. diet tonic (0) + 1 lime wedge & juice (3) = 99 calories!

Low Calorie Alcoholic Drink #2—Wine Spritzers

Diluting your drink will not only slow down your alcohol consumption, it will also keep you from piling on the calories. Wine spritzers are an easy, low-calorie choice that only require 2 ingredients. Guys may feel too manly for them, but ladies - now you can have your alcohol and drink it too!

Red Wine Spritzer: 5 fl. oz. of Merlot (120) + 2 fl. oz. sparkling water (0) = 120 calories!

Low Calorie Alcoholic Drink #3—Rum & Coke

When drinking a rum & Coke or some other whiskey & Coke, simply replacing that full calorie (& very sugary) cola with a diet alternative makes it a low-calorie alcoholic drink. You can shave off up to 100 calories per drink!

Low Calorie Alcoholic Drink #4—Highball

Traditionally, this drink is made with ginger ale, but requesting diet ginger ale shaves off 45 calories. This is one of the simplest low calorie alcoholic drinks to make: fill a highball glass with ice, 2 ounces whiskey and 4 fluid ounces of diet ginger ale. Mix, & enjoy for just 128 calories.

CHAPTER TWELVE
Recipes That Rock

Below you will find some yummy, easy and healthy recipes for you to try. Make them for yourself, make them for your family, friends, co-workers, the mail carrier- they'll all thank you!

Eggplant (or Chicken) Parmesan (which can be either lunch or dinner).

Note: Pine nuts replace the usual flour coating, adding crunchy texture and

nutty flavor. Serve with whole-wheat pasta (1/4 cup).

Makes 4 servings:

2 cups low-sugar pasta sauce

2 cups pine nuts, coarsely chopped

1/4 cup freshly grated Parmesan cheese

2 tsp dried Italian seasoning (or a combo of basil, rosemary and/or thyme)

1 pound eggplant (or chicken, or ½ & ½), about 1/3 inch thick

2 tsps extra-virgin olive oil

1/2 cup part skim mozzarella cheese, shredded

2 egg whites, beaten lightly

sea salt and freshly ground black pepper.

1. Heat oven to broil. Bring sauce to low simmer in a small saucepan over medium-low heat. Remove from heat and cover to keep warm.
2. Stir together pine nuts, Parmesan cheese and Italian seasoning in a wide, shallow dish. Dredge the eggplant slices in egg whites, then season the eggplant slices on both sides w/salt and pepper, then dredge both sides in the nut mixture, pressing to adhere.
3. Heat oil in large nonstick skillet over medium-low heat. Add eggplant and cook until coating is golden brown, about 3 minutes per side. If nuts brown too quickly, reduce heat.
4. Place eggplant slices in a baking pan, top evenly with mozzarella, and broil until cheese melts, about 30 seconds.
5. Spoon 1/2 cup of warm sauce on each plate, top with eggplant. Enjoy!

About 250-300 calories per serving.

Spinach Quiche

1 c. regular oats

1/4 c. oat bran

2 tbs chilled light tub margarine

1/4 c. cold water

1 c. chopped leeks

1 c. sliced mushrooms

1 c. evaporated non-fat milk or non-dairy substitute

1/3 c. Parmesan cheese

1/2 tsp sea salt

1/2 tsp dill

1/4 tsp black pepper

3 large egg whites

2 large eggs

1 10-oz package frozen chopped spinach, thawed & squeezed dry

1/2 c. shredded Swiss cheese

1. Preheat oven to 375. Spray 9-10" pie plate w/ cooking spray.
2. Prepare crust by combining oats and oat bran in medium bowl. Add margarine and cut in w/pastry blender or spatulas. Add water & stir until just moistened. Press dough evenly into prepared pie plate. Bake for 8 minutes or until lightly browned.
3. In the meantime, spray large skillet w/cooking spray and place over medium-high heat; add leeks and sauté for 5 minutes, reduce heat & simmer 5 minutes more; remove from heat.
4. Combine milk and next 7 ingredients in blender; process until smooth. Add leek mixture & stir well. Pour into pie crush and top w/shredded cheese.
5. Bake for 35 minutes or until set in center. Let stand for 5 minutes.

Makes 6 servings

Per serving: 240 calories, 15 g protein & 23 carbs, 4.5 g. fiber.

Serve with either a cup of roasted or fresh veggies and a dinner salad with 1-calorie spray-on dressing.

Braised chicken w/white beans & baby spinach

1 lb. chicken breasts

1/2 tsp dried thyme leaves, crushed

1/8 tsp ground black pepper

1-1/2 tsp light tub margarine

1 medium onion, finely chopped

3 cloves garlic, finely chopped

1-1/2 cups low fat, reduced sodium chicken broth

1/4 c. dry white wine or water

1 can (16 oz.) cannellini or white kidney beans, rinsed & drained.

1 bag (10 oz) baby spinach leaves

1. Season chicken w/thyme and pepper. Melt 1 tbsp margarine in 12-inch non-stick skillet over medium-high heat and cook chicken until brown, about 6 minutes. Remove chicken from skillet and set aside.

2. Add remaining 1/2 tbs margarine in same skillet & cook onion, stirring occasionally, 6 minutes or until tender. Add garlic and cook 30 seconds. Add broth and wine and bring to a boil over high heat.

3. Reduce heat to low and return chicken to skillet. Simmer covered for 4 minutes. Stir in beans and spinach. Simmer uncovered, stirring occasionally for about 5 more minutes or until chicken is thoroughly cooked.

Makes 4 servings (you can have leftovers for a lunch the next day, or halve
the recipe)

Calories: 260, Protein, 24 g.; carbs 23 g., fiber 7g

NOTE: you can substitute shrimp for the chicken if you wish

Side Dishes:

Sweet potato fries: halve a sweet potato, then slice into slivers. beat an egg white lightly, wash each fry in egg wash, put on foil-lined cookie sheet. Spray lightly with olive oil or cooking spray olive oil spray, then season (I use sea salt & ground pepper & garlic powder, you can get creative with whatever spices you like - the pumpkin pie spices are also nice, like nutmeg). You can sprinkle lightly with grated Parmesan too. Bake for about 15-20 mins at 400, then I broil for another minute to crisp them. You can have this as a side a few times a week. Enjoy! Sometimes I dip mine in a little non-fat plain yogurt just for a change.

Grill Recipes

Lean Steak and Mushroom Salad

2 tablespoons of your favorite steak seasoning

1 tablespoon extra-virgin olive oil

1 tablespoon white wine vinegar

2 teaspoons Dijon mustard

1 teaspoon lemon juice

1 teaspoon Worcestershire sauce

12 ounces boneless sirloin steak (2 inches thick), well trimmed

8 ounces fresh mushrooms, cleaned and sliced

1/2 cup green onions, sliced

1/4 cup fresh parsley, minced

1 cup cherry tomatoes, sliced

1. Whisk together extra virgin olive oil, white wine vinegar, Dijon mustard, lemon juice and Worcestershire sauce, set aside. (a low calorie dressing of your choice can be substituted)

2. Season both sides of steak. Cook steak on preheated grill until medium rare or desired doneness is reached, about 4-5 minutes per side. Slice into 1/4 in. thick slices.

3. Place mushrooms, green onions and fresh parsley in large bowl.

4. Add steak to mushroom mixture and toss with dressing. Garnish with cherry tomatoes and serve immediately.

   Makes four servings. Calories: 167, Total fat: 8.6 g

Grilled Portobellos Sauteed in Wine

4 portobello mushroom caps

1 tablespoon olive oil

1 tablespoon butter

1 shallot, thinly sliced

1 cup white wine

1. Preheat grill for high heat.
2. Place mushrooms onto the grill, smooth side up. Grill until they start to soften, about 10 minutes. Turn over, and grill on the other side for about 5 minutes.
3. Meanwhile, heat olive oil and butter in a large skillet over medium heat. Add the shallot, and saute for a few minutes, stirring frequently until the shallots are softened.
4. Remove mushrooms to a cutting board, and slice. Place into the skillet, and increase the heat to high. Cook for about a minute, and then pour in the wine. Continue to cook and stir until the wine is nearly evaporated. Remove from heat, and serve. Makes four servings. Calories: 145 Total Fat: 6.5g

Grilled Salmon or any other firm fish suitable for grilling

1 pound salmon fillets with the skin on

1 lemon cut in half

1 tablespoon dried dill weed

1/4 teaspoon garlic powder

sea salt to taste

freshly ground black pepper to taste

1. Preheat Grill. Squeeze the lemon on the salmon then Season salmon with dill, garlic powder, sea salt, and pepper.

2. Grill salmon about 5 or 6 minutes per side starting with the skin side down or until salmon is easily flaked with a fork. Remove the skin and serve.

Makes four servings. Calories: 220 Total Fat: 11g

Grilled chicken marinated in fat-free Italian dressing

4 skinless, boneless chicken breast halves

1 cup fat free Italian-style dressing

1. Wash chicken thoroughly.
2. Split individual breasts in half to make them thinner.
3. Place chicken breasts in large sealable bag. Add 1 cup fat-free Italian dressing and close. Let marinate for 5 to 10 minutes.
4. Grill chicken over medium heat.

Makes four servings. Calories: 248 Total Fat: 3.1g

As a side to any of these meals grill some vegetables.

Many veggies do well on the grill, but these are just made for it: asparagus, corn, eggplant, mushrooms, peppers (bell or hot), cherry tomatoes, yellow squash, zucchini, onions, even green beans.

The possibilities are endless. Remember, the more colorful the veggies on your plate, the more disease-fighting antioxidants you're consuming.

The easiest way to prep bell peppers is to cut them in half from top to bottom, remove stem and seeds, and then quarter each side.

For the asparagus and green beans, use foil on the grill or a grill basket.

When cooking small mushrooms, use a skewer or a grill basket.

Ingredients

Fresh Veggies of your choice

1 tablespoon olive oil

Garlic or any seasoning to taste

1. Preheat grill for high heat.
2. Lightly coat the vegetables with olive oil. Season to taste.
3. Grill over high heat for 2 to 3 minutes, or to desired tenderness.

Sweets & Treats

Chocolate-Chip Oatmeal Cookies

Using lowfat sour cream or yogurt in place of half the butter of regular chocolate chip cookies cuts the fat, and oatmeal gives them a great texture and taste!

1 c. unbleached white flour

1 c. whole wheat flour

1 ½ tsp. baking soda

1 tsp. salt

2 c. oats

½ c. butter or margarine

¾ c. brown sugar

¾ c. sugar

½ c. egg whites

3 tsp. vanilla

2/3 c. lowfat sour cream or lowfat plain yogurt

2 c. semisweet chocolate chips

1. Heat oven to 375.
2. Sift together dry ingredients.
3. In a large bowl, beat together butter and sugars, then mix in egg, vanilla and yogurt. Gradually mix dry ingredients into wet. Stir in chocolate chips.
4. Drop by rounded spoonfuls onto parchment-covered cookie sheets. Bake about 10 minutes. Makes 6 dozen. Also great with white chocolate chips and dried cranberries, or dark chocolate chunks and dried cherries.

Banana-Chocolate Chip Muffins

A family favorite! Using ripe bananas means you need less sugar than traditional muffin recipes.

1 c. unbleached white flour

2/3 c. whole wheat flour

1 tsp. baking powder

½ tsp. ground cinnamon

¼ tsp. salt

3 medium sized very ripe bananas

3 egg whites

¼ c. canola oil

¼ c. milk

1 tsp. vanilla

¾ c. mini semisweet chocolate chips

1. Heat oven to 375.
2. Sift together dry ingredients.
3. In large bowl, mash bananas, then stir in egg, oil, milk and vanilla.
4. Gradually stir in dry ingredients- do not overmix. Stir in chocolate chips.
5. Spray muffin cups with nonstick cooking spray; fill ¾ full. Bake for about 20 minutes (12 minutes for mini muffins). Makes 1 dozen regular or 2-3 dozen mini muffins.

Blueberry Cereal Muffins

The not-so-secret ingredient is blueberry cereal.

1 c. lowfat plain yogurt

¼ c. no-cholesterol egg product

¼ c. canola oil

¼ c. each white and brown sugars

2/3 c. unbleached white flour

2/3 c. whole wheat flour

1 tsp. baking soda

1 tsp. ground cinnamon

¼ tsp. salt

1 c. crushed blueberry cereal

1 c. fresh or frozen (do not thaw) blueberries

1. Heat oven to 375.
2. In large bowl, mix yogurt, egg, oil and sugars.
3. Stir in dry ingredients, including cereal. Do not overmix. Gently fold in blueberries.
4. Spray muffin cups with nonstick cooking spray; fill ¾ full. Bake for about 20 minutes (12 minutes for mini muffins). Makes 1 dozen regular or 2-3 dozen mini muffins.

Carrot Cake

This is a moist and delicious cake! Serve immediately or refrigerate as it does not keep long.

1 ¾ c. unbleached white flour

2/3 c. whole wheat flour

2 tsp. baking soda

2 tsp. cinnamon

1 tsp. pumpkin pie spice

¼ tsp. salt

1/2 c. egg whites

1 c. brown sugar

¼ c. canola oil

2/3 c. lowfat plain yogurt

3 c. shredded carrots

¾ c. golden raisins

1. Heat oven to 350.
2. Sift together dry ingredients.
3. Beat together egg, brown sugar, oil, and yogurt. Gradually mix in dry ingredients. Stir in carrots and raisins.
4. Spray a 9x13" pan or Bundt pan with cooking spray; flour lightly. Fill pan and bake for approximately 40-45 minutes. Serves 12-15.

AFTERWARD

Yay! You did it! Or you're going to –

No longer will you have to worry about eating anything other than a salad in public, only to go home and eat 2 ice cream bars…(remember – have a half of one, and save the other one and a half for another day – this is NOT a diet! It's a way of life)…

No more being embarrassed to tell a sales lady your real size when trying on clothes (aren't you sick of popping buttons off a too-small blouse in the dressing room, then slinking back to the girl, handing her your plastic number tag, acting as if nothing happened…) - you'll be able to try on and purchase your new, smaller size!

You won't have to put off invitations to events – not because you aren't dying to go, but because you can't stomach the thought of running into an ex-boyfriend you've not seen in forever, hoping he won't notice your added girth. Instead…you'll be raring to go, your only concern being which hot little number you're going to shimmy your new bod into!

You will offer to take your kids to the beach! You may even offer to take other people's kids to the beach, just so you can slip out of that cover-up to reveal the new you! Ok, let's not get carried away – your own kids are a handful enough. Still, you get the picture.

You will at long last be proud of yourself, of who you've become, inside and out, and you'll never have to lose weight again…remember, this is a plan for life – yours. Don't you deserve it?

A licia Hunter, 44, has transformed personal loss into a thriving career as a celebrity beauty and lifestyle expert. She got her start by putting make-up on any sibling who would sit still long enough, and ever since then, all she's ever wanted to do is help people look and feel beautiful! She has launched her own business by offering services as a personal weight loss consultant and as an eyelash extension artist. Alicia divides her time between south Florida, where she lives with her two children, and New York City.

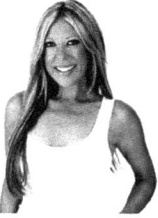

A my Hunter-Dutta has been writing for roughly three decades, and she hopes she's come a long way since her first novel, completed in sixth grade, entitled *The Adventures of Ernie Ohsoweird.* As a stay-at-home mom, she's maintained her sanity mostly through writing and the occasional glass of wine. Last year, her short story *A Christmas Tale* won the Rogues Gallery Writer's contest, and was subsequently published in the anthology *Writing Is Easy* (ClearView Press, Inc.). Ms. Hunter-Dutta is currently seeking agent representation of her mystery novel *The Time of Your Life (Unless You Die First...),* available on the Amazon and Barnes & Noble websites.

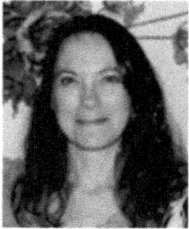

Lightning Source UK Ltd.
Milton Keynes UK
UKHW020802021022
409789UK00008B/51

9 781935 795889